THE **NURSE MANAGER'S**
LEGAL COMPANION
A **Practical Guide** to **Best Legal Practices**

DINAH BROTHERS, RN, JD

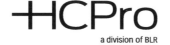
HCPro

a division of BLR

The Nurse Manager's Legal Companion is published by HCPro, a division of BLR.

Copyright © 2015 HCPro, a division of BLR

Download the additional materials of this book at *www.hcpro.com/downloads/12432*

ISBN: 978-1-55645-814-9

HCPro provides information resources for the healthcare industry.

HCPro is not affiliated in any way with The Joint Commission, which owns the JCAHO and Joint Commission trademarks. MAGNET™, MAGNET RECOGNITION PROGRAM®, and ANCC MAGNET RECOGNITION® are trademarks of the American Nurses Credentialing Center (ANCC). The products and services of HCPro are neither sponsored nor endorsed by the ANCC. The acronym "MRP" is not a trademark of HCPro or its parent company.

Dinah Brothers, RN, JD, Author
Claudette Moore, Editor
Erin Callahan, Vice President, Product Development & Content Strategy
Elizabeth Petersen, Executive Vice President, Healthcare
Matt Sharpe, Production Supervisor
Vincent Skyers, Design Services Director
Vicki McMahan, Sr. Graphic Designer
Jason Gregory, Layout/Graphic Design
Tyson Davis, Cover Designer

Advice given is general. Readers should consult professional counsel for specific legal, ethical, or clinical questions.

Arrangements can be made for quantity discounts. For more information, contact:

HCPro
100 Winners Circle Suite 300
Brentwood, TN 37027
Telephone: 800-650-6787 or 781-639-1872
Fax: 800-785-9212 Email: *customerservice@hcpro.com*

Visit HCPro online at *www.hcpro.com* and *www.hcmarketplace.com*

Contents

About the Author

Dinah Brothers, RN, JD, is a nurse attorney based in Texas. Brothers is a solo practitioner specializing in civil litigation. In her practice, she defends healthcare professionals in civil and administrative proceedings.

Prior to becoming an attorney, Brothers worked as a nurse for 10 years. Her nursing experience includes psychiatric nursing, nursing management, and nursing education.

Acknowledgments

My heartfelt appreciation is extended to the editorial staff at HCPro. I specifically want to thank Claudette Moore, whose professional work ethic made this experience very rewarding and enjoyable.

Book Resources

All the book's resources are available to download and customize for your practice. To access the resources, please visit: *www.hcpro.com/downloads/12432.*

Nursing Continuing Education

Nursing contact hours

HCPro is accredited as a provider of continuing nursing education by the American Nurses Credentialing Center's Commission on Accreditation.

You will find complete information about earning 3 hours of Continuing Nursing Education credits, as well as instructions on how to take the continuing education exam, on our website. Please visit *www. hcpro.com/downloads/12432* to access the Nursing Education Instructional Guide for this educational activity.

Disclosure statement

The planners, presenters/authors, and contributors of this CNE activity have disclosed no relevant financial relationships with any commercial companies pertaining to this activity.

Educational Objectives

1. Define the role of the nurse manager
2. Discuss the legal definition of the standard of care

3. Distinguish between negligence and professional malpractice

4. Identify protected persons under Title VII

5. Describe the legal components of the Americans with Disabilities Act

6. Define the purpose of the Family Medical Leave Act

7. Describe the five major steps in the hiring process

8. Evaluate a job applicant's qualifications within the boundaries of the law

9. Discuss when job descriptions must be updated on your unit

10. List the purposes of policies and procedures

11. Define the duty of the nurse manager in enforcing policies and procedures

12. Discuss how hospital policies and procedures are applied in court

13. Explain the legal significance of the yearly employee evaluation

14. Explain the four steps of progressive discipline

15. Implement the termination process in a confidential and respectful manner

16. Discuss conscientious objection

17. Discuss the impact of violence against nurses

18. Explain reasons for violence in the workplace

19. Discuss the nurses legal duty to report illegal and unsafe practices

20. Discuss how the nurse manager may contribute to retaliation against employees

21. Understand forms of retaliation which a whistleblower may experience

22. Identify the liability risks associated with inadequate staffing

23. Explain the nurse manager's responsibility for agency nurses

24. Define patient abandonment in the context of inadequate staffing

25. Define nursing delegation

26. Discuss the role of the nurse manager and the charge nurse in delegation

27. Enumerate the principles of delegation

28. Discuss the expectation of privacy in regards to social media

29. Enumerate examples of social media misuse

30. Discuss the "no tolerance" policy of social media misuse

31. Discuss the importance of teamwork in healthcare delivery

32. List the four core competencies of interprofessional collaboration

33. Identify the role of communication in interprofessional collaboration

34. Discuss the reasons to purchase professional liability insurance

35. Identify three actions a nurse must take when appearing before the disciplinary panel of a state nursing board

Introduction

Nurse managers serve a very important role in the healthcare field; achieving the position of nurse manager signifies that hospital management recognizes your professionalism, leadership, and contribution to nursing. As a nurse manager, your professional responsibilities increase significantly, and you are held to a different level of accountability. To be successful as a nurse manager and to avoid legal issues, you must understand what is expected of you in that role and comprehend the legal risks that come with the job.

Nurse managers often have little to no management training, but they are expected to operate within the law and will be held legally accountable should they fail to do so. The purpose of this book is to examine the common legal risks nurse managers face and to provide them with practical skills they can use to minimize those risks. We will discuss the law and legal standards for nurse management, risk reduction behaviors, and tools that the nurse manager can implement with specific legal examples.

On the first page of each chapter, you'll notice an excerpt from a typical nurse manager job description. You'll see that these definitions of the nurse manager's professional responsibilities are directly tied to the legal risks explored in each chapter.

What You Will Find in This Book

Every nurse manager must be well versed in employment law and in how to approach employment issues within the bounds of state and federal law. Employment law is lengthy, detailed, and often difficult. This book boils down complicated employment law and defines the employment law "must knows" for the nurse manager, including all aspects of human resource management.

Interviewing, hiring, and maintaining staff is a primary responsibility of the nurse manager, but it must be done in compliance with the law. This book discusses the legal aspects of interviewing, hiring, and orienting new staff and the legal ramifications for failing to do so. It also addresses the difficult decision to terminate an employee and how to do so legally and respectfully.

Nursing issues, such as safety in the workplace, unit staffing, and delegation and supervision, have specific, and increased, liability risks for the nurse manager. We will discuss these issues from the nurse manager's point of view, identifying liability risks and risk management techniques to incorporate into daily practice. We will examine the liability risk of social media use and how the nurse manager should respond when off-duty nursing staff violate social media policies. The nurse as whistleblower has been given much media attention lately, so we have dedicated a chapter to that topic, providing the nurse manager with guidelines for protecting whistleblowers from retaliation.

Above all, nurse managers must be proactive about protecting their nursing licenses. Your nursing license is a property right, and you must treat it as such. We insure everything important to us—our homes, our cars, our vacations—and our nursing licenses should be insured as well. Even when nurse managers do everything correctly in their nursing practice, they can still be sued or called before their state licensing board. This book discusses the steps to take should such an issue arise.

At the very end of this book, you'll find a short chapter presenting 10 strategies that nurse managers should practice daily to reduce the risk of liability and to support their roles as respected nursing leaders. For nurse managers facing the challenging and rewarding tasks of ensuring that patient care on their units is delivered in a safe, effective, and legal manner, we hope you will find this book to be a trusted source of support.

1

The Legal Environment of Nursing Management

Nurse Manager Job Description

The nurse manager advocates for patient health by developing day-to-day management and long-term planning of the assigned unit, directing and developing human resources, collaborating with interprofessional teams, and maintaining the standard of care.

Learning objectives

After reading this chapter, the participant will be able to do the following:

- Define the role of the nurse manager
- Discuss the legal definition of the standard of care
- Distinguish between negligence and professional malpractice

With the increased responsibility accorded to your role as nurse manager comes added legal accountability for your work and your team. To be successful in avoiding legal issues, you must understand what is expected of you and how to meet those expectations within the realm of the law. This book as a whole gives you the "must knows" for minimizing legal risk; in this chapter, we explore the underpinnings of the legal environment for nursing management.

The Role of Nurse Manager

As a nurse manager, you are responsible for directing, organizing, and supervising the work of the hospital nursing staff assigned to your unit. The staff typically includes registered nurses, licensed vocational/practical nurses, nursing assistants/orderlies/aides, and medical clerks/secretaries. The nurse manager usually reports to the chief nursing officer, director of nursing, or vice president of nursing, although there is some variation depending upon the setting and its governance.

Your role as nurse manager is very important, and you must be adequately prepared to meet your obligations; you represent "on-the-floor" hospital administration and are the first line of defense in ensuring that patient care delivery is within the standard of care. Nurse managers are "critical in the provision of high-performing effective and efficient care in the patient care delivery setting" (Chase, 2010).

As a nurse manager, you are responsible for the day-to-day management and clinical care delivered on your assigned unit. You're expected to be competent in a number of skills and behaviors, including but not limited to the following:

- Human resource management, including interviewing, hiring, and disciplinary actions
- Quality improvement and risk management
- Maintaining the competency of nursing staff
- Financial and budget management
- Interprofessional collaboration and communication
- Ensuring that patient care is delivered within the standard of care

As stated earlier, newly minted nurse managers frequently have little or no management training before they assume their duties (Chase, 2010), but they are still expected to operate within the law and will be held legally accountable if they do not.

Experienced and new managers alike must place emphasis on two areas of concern—upholding the standard of care in nursing practice and following established policies and procedures.

The Standard of Care in Nursing Practice

Nurses are expected to be competent to provide patient care and to deliver that care within the scope of their defined practice. When a nurse fails to provide competent care in his or her particular specialty or practices outside the scope of practice, that nurse may be found liable for violating professional nursing standards and may be held legally accountable.

When the quality of a nurse's professional practice is at issue, one of the first questions asked is whether he or she practiced within the standard of care. The *standard of care* is a set of minimal competencies that a nurse must possess and practice to provide acceptable care. In *King v. State of Louisiana*, 728 So.2d 1027, 1030 (La. App. 1999), the court defined the standard of care as follows:

> *A nurse who practices her profession in a particular specialty owes to her patients the duty of possessing the degree of knowledge or skill ordinarily possessed by members of her profession actively practicing in such specialty under similar circumstances. It is the nurse's duty to exercise the degree of skill ordinarily employed, under similar circumstances, by members of the nursing profession in good standing who practice their profession in the same specialty and to use reasonable care and diligence, along with his/her best judgment, in the application of his/her skill to the case.*

The standard of care has been further defined as the *reasonably prudent nurse standard,* or what a nurse with similar experiences and education would do in similar circumstances.

Standard of care example

Evaluating how courts have applied this standard clarifies the legal expectations of the standard of care. For example, in *Sabol v. Richmond Height General Hospital,* 676 N.E.2d 958 (Ohio App. 1996), Mr. Sabol was admitted to the intensive care unit of a general acute care hospital following an overdose suicide attempt. The unit's intent was to stabilize Mr. Sabol while arrangements were made to transfer him to a psychiatric facility. While in intensive care, however, Mr. Sabol became increasingly paranoid and delusional.

The nursing staff discussed the steps that should be taken to calm the patient and decided against the use of restraints, fearing that they would increase Mr. Sabol's agitation. Instead, in an attempt to calm the patient, a nurse remained at Mr. Sabol's bedside. Mr. Sabol got out of bed, knocked down the nurse in his room, fought past two other nurses, and ran off the intensive care unit. Once off the unit, Mr. Sabol knocked out a third-story window and jumped, fracturing his arm and sustaining other minor injuries.

The *Sabol* Court held that the intensive care nurses were not liable for Mr. Sabol's injuries. According to the court, the nurses realized that the patient was a threat to himself and had acted reasonably under the circumstances. The actions taken were fully consistent with basic professional standards of practice for medical-surgical nurses in an acute care facility. According to the *Sabol* Court, these nurses did not have, nor were they expected to have, specialized psychiatric nursing skills, and they would not be judged as though they did.

THE BOTTOM LINE

The *King* and *Sabol* decisions reassure nurses because the standard established is one of reasonableness: That is, nurses will be held accountable within their specialty area but will not be expected to possess knowledge and skills outside their specific area of practice.

Establishing the standard of care

In nursing, the standard of care is established through several channels, including research, state authorities, and professional associations. First, through research, the profession of nursing works to develop a foundation of knowledge upon which nursing care is delivered. Standards are also established by state authorities, such as state nursing boards. Such boards write laws and rules that dictate the scope of practice for nurses and govern the nurse's duty to patient care. There are also numerous state and national professional associations that define the standard of care.

As a nurse manager, you need to be aware of how and where the standard of care is defined, and you must understand the expectations of those standards. In a lawsuit related to standard of care, both parties (the one who initiated the proceeding and the one against whom the suit was brought) will call nursing professionals to establish the standard of care. These nurses are considered expert witnesses, meaning that they are authorities for the practice area in question and can speak to the knowledge and skills necessary to perform competently. These witnesses will give an opinion regarding whether the nurse on trial practiced within the standard of care.

Negligence in nursing

When a nurse fails to practice within the standard of care or practices outside the scope of his or her identified practice, that nurse may be sued for negligence. *Negligence* is defined as "conduct which falls below the standard established by law for the protection of others against unreasonable risk or harm." (Restatement [Second of Torts §282 1965). Therefore, when any person, regardless of professional status, is careless or fails to exercise reasonable conduct and another is injured, the acting party may be held negligent. Note that negligence may occur when a person acts or *fails to act* when a reasonably prudent person would have taken action in a similar situation.

Five elements must be established to hold a person liable for negligence:

1.   A duty of care owed by the defendant (the person sued in a civil proceeding) to the plaintiff (the party who brings the civil suit in a court of law)
2.   A breach of that duty
3.   An actual causal connection between the defendant's conduct and the resulting harm
4.   Proximate cause, which questions whether the harm was foreseeable
5.   Damages resulting from the defendant's conduct

Each of the five elements must be established in order to hold a person liable for negligence.

Professional malpractice

Professional malpractice is negligence committed by a professional person. A person may be found liable for professional malpractice when, acting within their professional capacity, they fail to exercise reasonable conduct. The standard for establishing professional malpractice is effectively the same as that for establishing negligence. When applied to nursing, the five elements of professional malpractice may be analyzed in the following case.

Professional malpractice example

In *Dent v. Memorial Hospital of Adel,* 509 S.E.2d 908 (Ga, 1998), a 15-month-old child was admitted to the hospital after being successfully resuscitated when he stopped breathing at home. The physician ordered the child to be placed on a pediatric apnea monitor. Although the patient was placed on the monitor, the nursing staff failed to activate the alarm. When the child stopped breathing, the alarm did not sound a warning, and the child died. The *Dent* Court found the nurse negligent and therefore liable for professional malpractice for failing to turn on the pediatric apnea monitor.

The standards of negligence applied to the *Dent* case would be analyzed as follows:

1. **Was there a duty of care owed by the defendant to the plaintiff?**

   Yes. The professional duty of the nurse was activated when he/she assumed care of the pediatric patient.

2. **Was there a breach of that duty?**

   Yes. The nurse had a duty to provide competent nursing care to the patient. A competent pediatric nurse in similar circumstances would have activated the pediatric apnea monitor. The duty to provide competent nursing care was breached when the nurse failed to do so.

3. **Was there an actual causal connection between the defendant's conduct and the resulting harm?**

   Yes. There was a causal connection between the defendant's failure to activate the pediatric apnea monitor and the plaintiff's death. It could be successfully argued that, but for the nurse failing to activate the apnea monitor, the patient would not have died.

4. **Were the defendant's actions the proximate cause of the plaintiff's injuries? Was it foreseeable that the plaintiff would sustain such injuries?**

   Yes. It was foreseeable that the failure to activate the pediatric apnea monitor (especially in a pediatric patient with previous apnea episodes) would cause the plaintiff to sustain such injuries and resulting death. It could be successfully argued by the plaintiff's attorney that the defendant's actions were the proximate cause of the plaintiff's death.

5. **Was the plaintiff damaged from the defendant's conduct?**

   Yes. The defendant's conduct caused damage to the plaintiff.

Here, all elements have been established to hold the nurse liable for professional negligence or professional malpractice.

The significant element in *Dent* is that a prudent nurse who was practicing within the standard of care would have activated the alarm for the pediatric patient, and the nurse who failed to do so was negligent and therefore liable for professional malpractice. Again, when a nurse is sued for professional malpractice, that nurse's professional actions will be compared to how a prudent and competent professional would have responded in a similar situation.

Nursing is defined by a set of specialized skills, knowledge, and abilities, and the law requires that nursing professionals practice within these established professional standards. Practicing outside the established professional standard of care constitutes professional malpractice.

Nurse Manager's Liability for Patient Care

One of a nurse manager's greatest concerns is that he or she may be held liable if a patient is injured due to staff nurse negligence. This is a valid concern: In some situations, nurse managers may indeed be held liable for a staff nurse's actions; in others, the liability lies with the hospital.

Respondeat superior

In law, the doctrine of *respondeat superior,* or vicarious liability, is based on the premise that employers are liable for the negligent acts of employees. Hospitals and other healthcare providers are engaged in the business of providing healthcare to the public, and it is the duty of that healthcare facility to hire competent, skilled employees to deliver that care. Therefore, when a nurse who is employed by a specific hospital is found to be negligent, the employing hospital may also be assigned liability, because the nurse's negligent act occurred within the scope of employment.

As a nurse manager, you are not held liable under the *respondeat superior* doctrine because you are not the employer of the negligent staff nurse. However, there are other ways that liability may be assigned to the nurse manager. For example, a nurse manager who fails to delegate nursing tasks within the standard of care may be held liable for negligent delegation.

Additionally, even though you are the nurse manager, there may be times you are required to provide direct patient care on your unit. In such situations, remember you are held to the reasonably prudent nurse standard and you will be held liable if the care you provide a patient is below the standard of care.

THE BOTTOM LINE

Knowing the legal risks of nurse managers will allow you to "play defense" and reduce the potential of legal liability.

References

Chase, L.K. (2010). *Nurse Manager Competencies* (Doctoral dissertation). Retrieved from Iowa Research Online. http://ir.uiowa.edu/etd/2681/

2

Employment Law
for the Nurse Manager

Nurse Manager Job Description

The nurse manager operates within state and federal law when completing
human resource management duties.

Learning objectives

After reading this chapter, the participant will be able to do the following:

- Identify protected persons under Title VII
- Describe the legal components of the Americans with Disabilities Act
- Define the purpose of the Family Medical Leave Act

Employment law is complicated, and it governs many of your duties as a nurse manager: Numerous state and federal laws define the legal rights of employees and affect the actions that employers may take. As a nurse manager, you are expected to have a basic understanding of employment law and adhere to it on a daily basis.

State and federal employment laws govern aspects of employment such as discrimination, disability, and medical leave, and numerous state and federal court decisions have interpreted these legal mandates. Today, employees are educated about their legal rights in the workplace, and they will take action against their employers if those rights are violated.

Each state has its own employment laws, so you must be familiar with the laws in the state where you practice. Most state laws are consistent with federal law; however, know that when a state law contradicts federal law, the state law is overridden and federal law is the ruling authority. Individual state laws will not be discussed here, but make sure that you know your state's employment law statutes.

In this chapter, we will focus on federal employment laws and discuss how these laws have been applied in legal and regulatory settings.

THE BOTTOM LINE

You will be held legally accountable if you violate employment law. If you have any questions regarding how to implement these laws, consult your human resources department. In your facility, the human resources department is your employment law specialist. If you have additional questions after meeting with them, consult with the legal department. However you get the information you need, make sure that you understand the law and how to apply it.

Illegal Discrimination

Because all workers deserve a fair opportunity to obtain and keep jobs, federal law prohibits discrimination in the workplace. Federal law specifically prohibits employment discrimination against workers on the basis of race, skin color, gender, religious beliefs, national origin, disability, or age.

Title VII of the Civil Rights Act of 1964

One of the most important anti-discrimination mandates is Title VII of the Civil Rights Act. Title VII is extensive and complicated. Here, a general overview of Title VII will be offered, with examples of how it has been applied in legal settings.

Under Title VII, it is illegal for an employer to make hiring decisions, promotions, terminations, or any other aspect of employment based upon the following:

1. Race

2. Color

3. Religion

4. Gender

5. National origin

In legal terms, people protected by Title VII are considered a "protected class." A *protected class* is defined as a group of people with common characteristics who are protected by statute (*Black's*, 2014). Under Title VII, it is illegal to discriminate against a person who is a member of a protected class. It's also illegal to discriminate against an individual because of his or her association with an individual who is a member of a protected class, as in the case of an interracial marriage.

Title VII violations occur when people in a protected class are treated differently from other employees in the workplace. For example, if a business that is legally mandated to operate within the confines of Title VII continuously fails to promote women within its organization, the business may be found to have discriminated against women. If challenged, the business must show that its promotion decisions were based on objective criteria and that the more qualified applicant always received the promotion.

Title VII also prohibits employer policies and practices that seem neutral but have a disproportionate impact on a given group of people. For example, a business can refuse to hire people who fail to meet a minimum height or weight requirement, but only if these physical requirements are clearly related to the physical demands of the particular job. The employer must have a valid business reason for such a policy, and if no business reason exists, then the employer may be violating Title VII.

Title VII is enforced by the Equal Employment Opportunity Commission (EEOC). Following investigation of a complaint, the EEOC will work toward a settlement agreement between the employer and the employee. Terms of such an agreement may require that the employee be reinstated in a job and/or that management and employees receive sensitivity training to avoid further discrimination in the workplace.

The EEOC will monitor compliance with the settlement agreement. If the parties are unable to reach one, then the EEOC will most likely issue the employee a "right-to-sue" letter. This letter allows the employee to proceed to federal court to sue the employer for violating his or her Title VII rights.

Finally, it is illegal to retaliate against an employee for filing a Title VII complaint.

➡ For details and examples of retaliation, see Chapter 7, "The Nurse as Whistleblower."

Title VII in court

To get a better understanding of the law, let's examine how Title VII has been applied in court and before the EEOC.

If you enforce a restriction, it must apply to everyone

The EEOC took action against a rehabilitation facility for discriminating against black and Caribbean employees. Official allegations stated that staff harassed black and Caribbean employees and allowed residents of the facility to make racially disparaging remarks to them. Additionally, the facility prohibited the use of Creole, the native language of the people in this protected class, but did not prohibit other non-English speaking staff from using their native languages. It was also alleged that stricter disciplinary rules were applied to the Creole-speaking employees than were applied to other employees. Finally, when the Creole-speaking employees complained about their treatment, staff retaliated against them.

The EEOC validated the discrimination claims, and the rehab facility entered into a settlement agreement with the EEOC to pay $900,000 dollars in damages, back pay, and attorneys' fees to the Creole-speaking staff (*EEOC v. William O. Benson Rehab Pavilion*, 1:05-cv-04601-NG-RER, filed April 20, 2007).

THE BOTTOM LINE

In your management career, you will be asked to make exceptions to a policy or do favors for employees. Remember, what you grant to one employee must be granted to all employees; otherwise, you run the risk of a discrimination claim. You must set professional boundaries and treat every employee in the same manner.

Hospital dress codes must accommodate religious attire

Title VII protects all aspects of religious practice, including religious icons, dress, and grooming practices. In its article "Religious Garb and Grooming in the Workplace: Rights and Responsibilities," the EEOC discusses steps that employers can take to ensure that they meet their legal responsibilities regarding religious freedom and dress (EEOC, n.d.).

In *EEOC v. Healthcare and Retirement Corp. of America d/b/a Heartland Health Care Center-Canton,* Case No. 07-13670 (E.D. Mich. Filed Aug. 21, 2007), discrimination allegations were substantiated when a nurse was terminated for wearing a kirpan, one of the sacred symbols of the Sikh religion, under her clothing. A kirpan is a dull knife with a blade three inches long; it is considered a symbolic sword to defend moral values and truth. The nurse wore this sheathed blade under her clothing as part of her religious conviction.

Upon learning that the nurse wore the kirpan at work, her supervisor told her that she could not continue to do so because it violated the facility's policies and procedures against weapons in the workplace. The nurse explained that Sikh code required her to wear the kirpan, provided literature on the subject, and showed him that the blade was no sharper than a butter knife.

When the nurse continued to wear the blade to work, she was terminated. She then filed a complaint with the EEOC, and it determined that she had been discriminated against based upon her religious convictions.

THE BOTTOM LINE

Hospital policies and procedures have strict dress codes that are in place to protect patients and staff. When a hospital accommodates an employee for a religious conviction, the dress code policy remains in full force and effect for other employees within the hospital. Hospital employees are expected to meet the dress code of a facility unless an accommodation has been requested and granted for a legally protected reason.

Patient privacy rights trump equal employment opportunities

In *Slivka v. Camden-Clark Memorial Hospital,* 594 S.E.2d 616 (W.Va 2004), a male nurse filed a discrimination lawsuit when a hospital refused to employ him as a nurse in the obstetrical department. As a registered nurse with obstetrical experience, Mr. Slivka was qualified for the position. His previous experience included assisting in the delivery room and working in three areas of a hospital's obstetrical services, including labor and delivery, postpartum, and the nursery. In reaching its hiring decision, the hospital stated that it would not consider a male nurse for obstetrics, citing concerns for patient privacy, staffing, and quality of care.

The hospital's obstetrics nurse manager provided an affidavit that established hospital policy. The nurse manager addressed the fact that all obstetrical patients are female and that obstetric care involved viewing, touching, and performing care to the patients' vaginal and perineal areas. The nurse manager stated that, in her personal experience with male student nurses, approximately 80% of obstetrical patients refused care from a male.

In reaching its decision, the *Slivka* Court researched relevant state and federal court decisions, and it concluded that a blanket prohibition against hiring males for jobs involving intimate personal care of female patients was discriminatory. However, court cases uniformly hold that patients have the right to ask for and receive care from a same-gender caregiver when intimate personal care is necessary—that is, a female patient does not have to accept intimate care from a male caregiver. The *Slivka* Court held that gender discrimination may be valid when patient privacy interests trump equal employment opportunities.

THE BOTTOM LINE

A patient has the right to refuse care from a person of the opposite gender. If the patient expresses discomfort with the gender of the staff caring for him or her, changing the staffing assignment is appropriate and is not discriminatory.

Pregnancy discrimination

In 1978, Title VII was amended with legislation that prohibits discrimination based upon pregnancy. (See the Pregnancy Discrimination Act of 1978.) Under Title VII, it is discrimination to base employment decisions upon a woman's pregnancy, childbirth, or related medical conditions. Women who are pregnant must be treated in the same manner as other similar job applicants or employees, which means that an employer cannot refuse to hire or promote a woman because of her pregnancy (or related condition) as long as she is able to perform the functions of the job.

Age discrimination

The Age Discrimination in Employment Act (ADEA) protects persons over the age of 40. Age discrimination occurs when a person who is older than 40 is treated less favorably due to his or her age. For example, comments or offensive remarks concerning a person's age may create a hostile work environment for that person and are prohibited by the ADEA.

In *Woody v. Covenant Health,* Docket No. 11-CV-62 (E.D. Tenn., May 8, 2013), the nurse manager posted a flyer and made verbal statements that she was looking to promote "Young Rising Stars" on her unit. At the time that the flyers were posted, all the current charge nurses were older than 40 years of age, placing them in a protected class.

The nurse manager told the existing charge nurses that their nursing positions were being eliminated, that a new job description would be written, and that the current charge nurses would have to reapply for their jobs. A nurse younger than 40 then began telling others on the unit that he was going to be the new charge nurse for the night shift. Nursing management did promote him to that position, and the nurse who had previously held the position, who was over 40, was forced to take a position with lesser pay and responsibility.

This case held that the rewritten job description was a pretext for discrimination. Based on the evidence that the new, younger charge nurse had been preselected to the position and that the job duties in the rewritten job description were basically the same as those in the original job description, the *Woody* Court held that the nursing supervisor had discriminated against the charge nurses based upon their ages.

THE BOTTOM LINE

Simple teasing or joking with employees about their age is not prohibited by law, but it can be a very slippery slope—it is difficult to determine where simple teasing ends and harassment begins. Harassment is illegal when it is so frequent or severe that it creates a hostile work environment or when it results in an adverse employment decision.

The Americans with Disabilities Act

People with disabilities have the right to work. The Americans with Disabilities Act (ADA) makes it illegal to discriminate against a person based upon that person's disability.

Like the Civil Rights Act of 1964, the ADA is an extensive and complicated law. Here, we will discuss some of the basic principles of the law that you are expected to understand and implement in your practice as a nurse manager.

The ADA defines a disabled person as someone who has a physical or mental impairment that substantially limits one or more major life activities, has a record of being substantially limited, or is regarded as being substantially limited. Such conditions include but are not limited to deafness, blindness, intellectual disability, partially or completely missing limbs, mobility impairments requiring the use of a wheelchair, autism, cancer, cerebral palsy, diabetes, epilepsy, human immunodeficiency virus (HIV) infection, multiple sclerosis, muscular dystrophy, major depressive disorder, bipolar disorder, post-traumatic stress disorder, obsessive compulsive disorder, and schizophrenia.

The preceding list is not exclusive and, according to the ADA, other health conditions may be defined as disabilities on a case-by-case basis.

Physical or mental impairments that limit major life activities

According to the ADA, a physical impairment is any disorder, condition, cosmetic disfigurement, or anatomical loss affecting any part of the body. A mental impairment is any mental or psychological disorder. However, just suffering from a physical or mental impairment does not guarantee that a person is covered under the ADA. The impairment also must "substantially limit" one or more major life activities—defined as walking, speaking, breathing, performing manual tasks, seeing, hearing, learning, working, and sitting—of the affected person. An ADA determination is based on whether the impairment "substantially limits" major life activities.

Reasonable accommodations

The ADA recognizes that some people with disabilities may need "reasonable accommodations" so that they may complete job requirements. A reasonable accommodation is defined as follows:

> An adjustment made in a system to accommodate or make fair the same system for an individual based on a proven need (Black's, 2014).

Examples of a reasonable accommodation include, but are not limited to, special/additional equipment that allows the person to perform the job, scheduling changes, and work assignment changes. If a person is qualified for the position or is able to complete the responsibilities of the position with reasonable accommodation, then an employer must treat that person just as it treats all other applicants and employees; failure to do so violates the ADA.

Undue hardship

Employers are required by law to make reasonable accommodations in the workplace, but those accommodations are not required if the accommodation places "undue hardship" on the employer. An *undue hardship* is defined as an accommodating action that places significant difficulty or expense on an employer (ADA National Network, n.d.). The determination of whether an accommodation presents undue hardship is made on a case-by-case basis. Some factors that contribute to the decision include the expense of the accommodation, the employer's resources, and the nature of the employer's organization. If a particular accommodation would result in undue hardship to the employer, then the employer must identify another accommodation that would not be such a hardship.

In nursing, when making the determination of undue hardship for a reasonable accommodation, consider factors such as patient acuity, patient safety, and nurse staffing numbers.

Hospitals are required to make only reasonable accommodations

Systemic lupus erythematosus (lupus) is recognized under the ADA as an employment disability. In *Willett v. State of Kansas,* 942 F.Supp. 1387 (D. Kan., 1996), a nurse who had been diagnosed with lupus was given reasonable accommodation so that she could continue her employment. The reasonable accommodations included providing the nurse with a lighter medication cart and assigning the nurse to a floor where less walking was required. Nonetheless, the nurse began to miss work frequently because she was having pain in her hands and back, and her knees were swelling. After the nurse was terminated for her frequent absences, she sued her employer, claiming that she was protected by the ADA.

The *Willet* Court ruled that frequent absences by a member of the nursing staff did impose an undue hardship on the facility and that the facility did not have the legal duty to accommodate such absences. The court recognized that even though lupus is a recognized disability under the ADA, only reasonable accommodations were required for this disability. The court acknowledged that each time the nurse called in and missed work, she forced the facility to face an undue hardship because the facility was still required to provide patient care even though the facility was short-staffed.

THE BOTTOM LINE

If an employee requests a reasonable accommodation for a disability, pay close attention to how that accommodation will impact patient care. If it negatively impacts patient care or causes safety issues on your unit, then you have a strong argument that the accommodation is an undue hardship. Make sure to consult your human resources department when an undue hardship is requested.

Must be qualified for the job

When a person who is covered under the ADA applies for a job, that person is protected under the ADA only if he or she is a qualified candidate. An employer is not legally required to place a person in a job for which the person is not qualified. Likewise, an employee who receives a reasonable accommodation from his or her employer must still perform the essential functions of the job and meet performance expectations defined in the job description. Whether applying for or currently holding a job, a person is protected under the ADA only if he or she has a disability *and* is qualified for a certain position.

Employees have taken extensive legal actions against their employers under the ADA. Next, we will examine some of those legal actions so that you may gain a better understanding of the legal environment in the workforce.

Reasonable accommodation does not require hiring an unqualified candidate

In *Hedrick v. Western Reserve Care System,* 355 F.3d 444 (6th Cir., 2004), a nurse fell, fractured her knee, and took a medical leave of absence from work. The nurse's recovery was complicated by a preexisting condition of osteoarthritis, and the nurse's physician determined that she was unable to return to her job as a staff nurse because her injury prohibited her from completing the walking, bending, and lifting that the job required. The hospital offered the nurse an office position in patient referral and scheduling, but the nurse rejected it. On two separate occasions, she applied and was rejected for quality assurance and nurse case manager positions on the grounds that other applicants were more qualified for the positions. Ms. Hedrick was issued a right-to-sue letter from the EEOC and filed suit against the hospital under the ADA.

In its written opinion, the *Hedrick* Court applied the legal mandates of the ADA to the facts. The *Hedrick* Court examined the "reasonable accommodation" of a disabled individual. To be entitled to a reasonable accommodation, the individual must be both disabled and qualified for the position. In this case, the court concluded that Western Reserve Care System did not violate the ADA by hiring other applicants that were more qualified than Ms. Hedrick for the quality assurance and case manager positions.

The court opined that the accommodation must be reasonable. In this case, a reasonable accommodation meant offering Ms. Hedrick a suitable hospital position consistent with her medical restrictions. An employer is not required to provide an employee with a position for which that person is not qualified, displaces other employees, or violates other employees' rights just to make an accommodation available to a disabled employee. Furthermore, an employer does not have to create a new position for a disabled employee or train that person to fill a position for which he or she was not qualified before he or she requested reasonable accommodation for a disability.

A position offered as a reasonable accommodation must be as comparable as the employer can offer relative to the employee's prior position in terms of pay, benefits, and status. There is no requirement to promote a disabled employee to a better position just to fulfill the reasonable accommodation request. Therefore, Ms. Hedrick could not establish discrimination based on the fact that she was not offered the nurse case manager job: It was considered a promotion, and she was not the most qualified candidate.

Furthermore, the *Hedrick* Court stated that an employee does not have to accept any position that is offered as a reasonable accommodation. However, by turning down a legitimate reasonable accommodation, the employee forfeits the right to sue for disability discrimination under the ADA.

THE BOTTOM LINE

An employer does not have to offer the position that the employee wants—the requirement is that they offer one that is comparable in terms of pay, benefits, and responsibility.

The nurse manager must be aware of the disability

For a facility to provide reasonable accommodations for an employee, the facility must have been put on notice that the employee required such accommodations.

In *Webb v. Mercy Hospital,* 102 F.3d 958 (8th Cir., 1996), Diana Webb was receiving care from a physician for depression; however, she did not notify her nurse manager about her condition. Ms. Webb did present her nurse manager with a physician's note stating that Ms. Webb should not work nights due to fatigue. This request was accommodated by nursing management for a couple of months. Nursing management then asked Ms. Webb to begin taking night shifts again, but Ms. Webb refused.

Over the next several weeks, Ms. Webb's behavior became more erratic. She made statements that were threatening to other staff members. She verbalized that she understood why someone who had been in the news for killing people had done so, voicing veiled death threats to other employees.

Nursing management disciplined Ms. Webb for her disruptive and insubordinate behavior, and she was told that she must participate in the employee assistance program for counseling or she would be terminated. Ms. Webb refused, and she was terminated from her nursing position.

After having been terminated, Ms. Webb showed up at a staff meeting. She was very disruptive and agitated, and she refused to leave. The vice president of patient care was notified and instructed Ms. Webb to leave the hospital, but she continued to refuse to do so. Ultimately, Ms. Webb was removed by hospital security.

Ms. Webb sued the hospital under the ADA, claiming that she had been illegally terminated because of her disability. Although Ms. Webb was suing under the ADA, she had never given notice to nursing management that she was diagnosed with depression and needed reasonable accommodation to perform her job. The *Webb* Court determined that nursing management had no idea that Ms. Webb had been diagnosed with depression.

Ms. Webb's supervisors did testify that she was a difficult and insubordinate employee but, according to the court, that did not put nursing management on notice that she had a mental disability. Ms. Webb's case against the hospital was dismissed.

THE BOTTOM LINE

It is the duty of the employee to inform the employer of a disability and to provide written confirmation of that disability. An employer is not expected to "guess" that the employee has a disability and has no duty to make a reasonable accommodation if not notified of it.

Family Medical Leave Act

The last employment law that we will briefly discuss here is the Family Medical Leave Act (FMLA). FMLA entitles eligible employees to take unpaid, job-protected leave for specific family and medical reasons. This leave from work may include intermittent leave or a reduced work schedule.

Covered employees are entitled to 12 work weeks of leave in a 12-month period for the following reasons:

1. The birth of a child and to care for the newborn child within one year of birth
2. The placement with the employee of a child for adoption or foster care and to care for the newly placed child within one year of placement
3. To care for the employee's spouse, child, or parent who has a serious health condition
4. A serious health condition that makes the employee unable to perform the essential functions of his or her job
5. Any qualifying exigency arising out of the fact that the employee's spouse, son, daughter, or parent is a covered military member on "covered active duty"

Under FMLA, employees who take this leave remain covered under the employer's health insurance, and conditions remain the same as if the employee had not taken leave.

The significant definition here is "serious health condition," which is defined as an illness, injury, impairment, or physical or mental condition. There are numerous situations in which an employee may qualify, and they are discussed in detail in FMLA.

Medical certification is required to verify serious medical conditions

When an employee seeks to take medical leave under FMLA, the employer may request that the medical condition be verified by a healthcare provider. Under FMLA, a healthcare provider is a physician, podiatrist, dentist, clinical psychologist, chiropractor, nurse practitioner, nurse midwife, clinical social worker, or a Christian Science practitioner. An employee cannot diagnose his or her own medical condition, as was seen in *Criscitello v. MHM Services,* 2013 WL 4049724 (M.D. Pa., Aug. 9, 2013).

In *Criscitello v. MHM Services,* a psychiatric nurse who had previously held the position of director of nursing was counseled by her employers concerning her job performance and leadership skills on the unit. At the time that she received this counseling, Ms. Criscitello was working as the mental health unit director.

While employed, Ms. Criscitello made requests for FMLA, but her requests were denied. Ms. Criscitello was ultimately fired from her position, and she then sued her employer for having violated her rights under FMLA.

At issue was whether Ms. Criscitello had a serious medical condition. Ms. Criscitello had never presented her employer with any written verification from a healthcare provider that she had a serious medical condition. Instead, she argued that she had diagnosed herself with stress, insomnia, and stress-related dermatologic and gastrointestinal disorders. Ms. Criscitello held that she was qualified to make this diagnosis due to her training as a clinical nurse specialist and her training in cognitive behavioral therapy, biofeedback, and progressive muscle relaxation techniques.

The court, however, disagreed. It stated that Ms. Criscitello, "who was neither a doctor nor nurse practitioner at the time—claims to have diagnosed herself as suffering from anxiety and depression" (p. 11). The court found that Ms. Criscitello was not qualified to diagnose herself with these conditions. The court found that Ms. Criscitello did not have a valid serious health condition and, thus, that her FMLA rights had not been violated.

THE BOTTOM LINE

FMLA is for serious medical conditions, not to be used on a whim by employees. As stated in one court decision, "Congress did not intend for an employee to stand on his or her FMLA rights whenever a need for aspirin or cold tablets arose" (*Hayduk v. City of Johnstown,* 580 F.Supp. 2d 429, 460 [W.D. Pa. 2008]).

Job restoration
When an employee returns from FMLA leave, the employee must be restored either to his or her original job or to an equivalent job, which means virtually the same job in terms of pay, benefits, and other terms of employment.

Conclusion

Employment law exists to protect an employee's rights and to ensure that employers have defined standards for implementing those rights. Please know that we have only discussed the "tip of the iceberg"—you must become familiar with the many other state and federal laws that govern employment.

As you can see from this brief overview, employment law is extensive and can be both confusing and difficult to implement. Employment situations must be examined on a case-by-case basis, and the law must be applied to each individual's situation. As the nurse manager, you must operate within the confines of the law. You will be held legally accountable if you fail to do so.

References

ADA National Network (n.d.). What is considered an "undue hardship" for a reasonable accommodation. Retrieved from *https//adata.org/faq/what-considered-undue-hardship-reasonable-accommodation.*

Black's Law Dictionary (10th ed.). (2014).

EEOC (n.d.). Religious Garb and Grooming in the Workplace: Rights and Responsibilities. Retrieved from *www.eeoc.gov/eeoc/publications/qa_religious_grd_grooming.cfm.*

3

Hiring and Maintaining Competent Staff

Nurse Manager Job Description

The nurse manager maintains nursing staff by recruiting, selecting, orienting, and training nurses and auxiliary staff.

Learning objectives

After reading this chapter, the participant will be able to do the following:

- Describe the five major steps in the hiring process
- Evaluate a job applicant's qualifications within the boundaries of the law
- Discuss when job descriptions must be updated on your unit

One of the most important duties that a nurse manager has is hiring staff and ensuring their competency to practice nursing. Hiring quality, competent nursing staff ensures that competent care is being delivered and reduces legal liability risks. When done correctly, hiring is a time-consuming and detailed process in which the nurse manager must perform due diligence to ensure that each job candidate is qualified and competent.

The Hiring Process

There are five major steps in the hiring process:

1. Defining the job

2. Recruiting for the position

3. Reviewing applications

4. Interviewing applicants

5. Orienting the new employee

Defining the Job

The job description should outline the position's essential functions and communicate the skills necessary to complete them successfully. Use the job description to define the specific skills and abilities required on your unit so that you can reference it in an interview and use it to assess whether an applicant is qualified.

Depending on the size of your hospital, the human resources department will most likely maintain job descriptions, which limits your role in writing them. However, as a nurse manager, you must guarantee that the job descriptions are current and that they accurately reflect staff nurse duties and responsibilities.

When nursing roles change, job descriptions must be changed to reflect these updates. This requires that you review the job descriptions at least yearly to determine whether the essential functions and responsibilities listed in the job description are current and accurately identify the responsibilities of nurses on your unit.

Job descriptions must be updated under the following circumstances:

1. There are professionally recognized changes to the standard of care
2. New medical advancements are accepted and implemented in your facility
3. New technology is implemented in your facility
4. Policies and procedures that impact the nurse's role change
5. Job responsibilities change

To ensure that job descriptions are up to date, ask your nursing staff to review and provide feedback on those used by your unit. Current employees know what skills are needed to perform on the unit and will be able to evaluate the job description critically. First, distribute a copy of the relevant job description to your employees, and ask them to make comments and changes by a certain date. Then, evaluate the feedback you receive from your employees, and compare it with your own assessment of the job description criteria. If updates need to be made, share edits with your supervisor, and work with human resources to add the changes.

THE BOTTOM LINE

Communicate to your staff members that their opinions, ideas, and feedback are important. When you request feedback regarding the accuracy of their job descriptions, you ensure that the job descriptions match the jobs, but you also demonstrate that you're interested in their input.

Once the updated job description has been accepted, distribute the finalized version to your nursing staff. If the change in the job description requires new competencies to be demonstrated, ensure that nurses demonstrate those competencies at this time so that they are practicing within the standard of care established by the newly implemented job description.

Current employees must sign a document stating that they received a copy of the updated job description and that they understand that they will be evaluated under the most recent standard, from this date forward. Place this signed document in the employee's personnel file. Figure 3.1 provides a sample employee verification of an updated job description.

Figure 3.1 Verification of Updated Job Description

I, [insert name], have received a copy of the updated job description for Staff Nurse III at Gentry Valley Hospital, dated [insert mm/dd/yyyy].

As a Staff Nurse III at Gentry Valley Hospital, I understand that from this date forward I will be evaluated under the expectations of this job description. I have read the job description and understand the required performance expectations.

Signature _____

Date _____

Witness Signature _____

Recruiting for the Position

As with all phases of the hiring process, complete the advertising and recruiting process in a manner that does not raise any suspicions that the hospital excludes a group of people protected by federal or state law. Here, your best resource is your human resources department, which can guide you through the recruitment process.

➡ For more in-depth information on legal issues related to recruiting, see Chapter 2, "Employment Law for the Nurse Manager."

Reviewing applications

The job application provides your first contact with individual applicants and gives you a tool for comparing applicants' experience and abilities. The job application is a legal document through which the hospital can communicate basic terms and conditions of employment and gain the applicant's consent to complete reference checks. The job application should notify the applicant that providing false or misleading information when completing the job description is grounds for termination.

The job application is bound by employment law and may only collect data that does not have the potential to discriminate against an applicant. It must be a standardized form that collects only legal, job-related information from each applicant.

Case study: Legal grounds for termination

Marilyn interviews for a position as charge nurse for the second shift in the intensive care unit where you are the nurse manager. She indicates that she works in a progressive and technologically savvy intensive care unit in the largest city of your state. She signs the application, verifying that the information provided in the application is truthful. Because of the stellar qualifications she has listed on the job application, she is selected from among many skilled applicants.

Soon after Marilyn begins her job, problems arise. She doesn't have the knowledge or abilities she identified on her job application. As the nurse manager, you start to think that something isn't right. You investigate and learn that Marilyn misrepresented her credentials and abilities in the job application.

What is your recourse?

You have legal grounds to terminate Marilyn from her position immediately if the employment application, signed by Marilyn, contains the following statement:

"I certify that all the information provided by me in connection with my application is true and complete, and I understand that any misstatement, falsification, or omission of information may be grounds for refusal to hire or, if hired, immediate termination."

Make sure to check with your human resources department before you take action. Have the human resources department approve the termination.

Interviewing applicants

The interview provides an opportunity to sell the applicant on the job and to find out whether he or she possesses the skills necessary to complete it. First, start the interview by offering the applicant some information about your unit and the job—the duties, the patient type, severity of illness and acuity on the unit, and the hospital system as a whole. Sharing this information gives the applicant a general understanding of your organization and helps you focus your questions about his or her skills and abilities. Once you have shared information about the expectations of the job, begin to question the applicant to determine whether he or she has the ability to meet the job expectations.

Questioning applicants within the boundaries of the law

The interview process is complicated, and with an increased awareness of the law, you will be able to use lawful questioning to determine whether an applicant is a proper fit for your unit.

Prior to the interview, establish a set of written, objective questions that you ask all applicants. These questions should focus on the job duties and the applicant's skills, abilities, and experience. If you have any concerns about the legality of your interview questions, consult your human resources department for guidance. Also, take a look at the questions in Figure 3.2 to see some examples of what *not* to ask.

Figure 3.2 Don't Ask These Interview Questions

When it comes to drawing the line between what is and isn't appropriate to ask a job candidate, the parameters aren't always clear. Some of the interview questions listed here may seem perfectly innocent, but all of them are illegal. In a 2014 CareerBuilder survey, 20% of hiring managers indicated that they'd asked a question in a job interview only to find out later that it was illegal to ask. Here are some obvious and not-so-obvious questions that you are not permitted to ask:

1. What is your religious affiliation?
2. Are you pregnant?
3. What is your political affiliation?
4. What is your race, color, or ethnicity?
5. How old are you?
6. Are you disabled?
7. Are you married?
8. Do you have or plan to have children?
9. Are you in debt?
10. Do you drink socially or smoke?

Often, the legality of the question depends on how the interviewer asks it. For example, a number of hiring managers didn't know whether it was legal to ask the following:

1. **"When do you plan to retire?"** Asking candidates about their long-term goals is okay, but asking when they plan to retire is off the table.

2. **"Where do you live?"** Asking candidates where they live could be interpreted as a way to discriminate based on their location and is therefore illegal. Asking them whether they are willing to relocate, however, is okay.

3. **"What was the nature of your military discharge?"** Asking why a military veteran was discharged is illegal; however, asking what type of education, training, or work experience they received while in the military is not.

4. **"Are you a U.S. citizen?"** While it's okay to ask whether a candidate is legally eligible for employment in the U.S., it's not okay to ask about citizenship or national origin.

Source: CareerBuilder, *http://prn.to/1CzIUIX*

Interviewing all potential nursing staff from the same set of standardized, objective questions will reduce the risk that an applicant might complain of discrimination during the interview process. As you proceed through the interview, make brief notes summarizing the applicant's responses.

Each interview is different, and your standardized questions will elicit responses that either require non-standardized follow-up questions or discussion of hospital policies and procedures. Such deviation is perfectly acceptable, but when you gather or provide additional information, make sure that you do so legally.

Sometimes we as nurse managers can learn helpful lessons from situations in which numerous legal and ethical errors were made. The case that follows perfectly illustrates employment law during the interview session and is a cautionary tale to all.

Inappropriate interviewing questions

In the case of *Sada v. Robert F. Kennedy Medical Center,* 56 Cal. App. 4th 138 (1997), Rosalva Sada was a Mexican-born nurse who was a citizen of the United States. As a child, she had attended a Catholic school where she had been required to learn English, which she spoke with no accent. Ms. Sada was also fluent in Spanish. Ms. Sada had blonde hair and a light complexion.

Ms. Sada was an agency nurse who worked many shifts at Robert F. Kennedy Medical Center. In one instance when she was working at the medical center, a Hispanic patient complained to her that there were not enough Spanish-speaking nurses on the unit, which made it difficult for him to communicate his medical needs. Ms. Sada took this information to the nurse manager. The nurse manager replied, "Hispanics spend 20 to 30 years in this country and do not bother to learn English, but they can find those public offices where they can get food stamps and all kinds of public assistance" (56 Cal. App. 4th 146).

Later that year, Ms. Sada was interviewed for a full-time nursing position by the same nurse manager who had made the comment above. During the interview, the nurse manager asked Ms. Sada, "Where are you from?" When Ms. Sada replied that she was from Mexico, the nurse manager said, "Well, why don't you just go back to Mexico and work there?" The nurse manager then stated, "We're going to have to end this," and terminated the interview. Ms. Sada was not hired for the position (56 Cal. App. 4th 146).

Ms. Sada brought suit against the medical center, claiming that she had been discriminated against based upon her national origin. The *Sada* Court determined that Ms. Sada's civil rights had been violated.

THE BOTTOM LINE

When questioning an applicant, focus on job requirements and on your hospital's policies and procedures. If you find yourself wanting to ask an applicant a question that applies only to that applicant, consider that a red flag for a potentially discriminatory question. You still can attempt to secure the information, but do so legally.

Disability-related questions

During the interview, you may question an applicant to determine whether the applicant is able to perform specific job-related tasks, but you may not ask about the existence or nature of a disability. You may legally ask an applicant the following:

- Whether he or she can perform a specific task, such as carrying a heavy object, if the job description requires the employee to perform the task

- Whether he or she can satisfy the organization's attendance requirements

- Whether he or she has the certificates or licenses required by the job

---

Case study: Asking appropriate disability-related questions

Zack, who is missing a portion of his right hand (including three fingers), applies for a nursing position at South Star Medical. As the nurse manager, you interview Zack for a position that requires the employee to administer patient treatments and medications and to calibrate technological equipment precisely. You avoid asking Zack whether or how his disability would affect his patient care. Instead, you ask Zack whether he has a valid nursing license, and you educate Zack about the medication administration policy. You tell Zack that nurses in the unit must be able to operate very sensitive equipment. You then ask Zack whether he will be able to perform these job requirements.

Have you interviewed Zack within the bounds of the law?

Yes. First, you gathered information about Zack's professional credentials. Then, you educated Zack about the specific tasks the position requires and asked whether he could perform those tasks. You have questioned Zack within the bounds of the law.

Making the Job Offer

Although most job offers are made orally via the telephone, work with your human resources department to follow up every job offer with a written confirmation that details the key elements of the employment understanding. These key elements include the following:

- The title of the position being offered

- Starting date

- Starting salary

- Job benefits

- Reminder of at-will status if applicable per your state's law (see note below for more information)

Have the applicant sign this understanding of employment, and maintain a copy of the document in the employee's file. This signed document provides clear proof that the employee accepted the terms of the employment agreement and can reduce your liability if employment issues arise. Use Figure 3.3, the sample employment offer letter, to draft a similar letter for your nursing unit. As always, have your human resources department review and approve the letter.

Figure 3.3 Sample Employment Offer Letter

January 1, 2016

Dear Nurse Jones,

I am pleased to offer you a full-time position as Staff Nurse III at West Lake Hospital. Your starting salary will be $35.00 per hour. You will work the 3 p.m.–11 p.m. shift, and you will receive a $2.50 per hour shift differential. You will receive a $4.50 per hour shift differential for weekend hours worked.

Please review the enclosed employee handbook. The handbook defines the current policies and procedures for employment at West Lake Hospital and details your job benefits, including medical coverage, paid vacation, and sick leave. It also describes your job responsibilities as Staff Nurse III. No one at West Lake Hospital is authorized to make oral commitments regarding employment, now or in the future.

If this offer of employment is acceptable to you, please sign a copy of this letter and return it to me within five days. I look forward to welcoming you as a member of our staff.

Sincerely,

Signature: _____

[insert name], Nurse Manager

I accept your offer of employment and acknowledge that I received a copy of your current employee handbook. I understand that my employment is at-will and that either you or I can terminate my employment at any time, for any reason. No oral commitments have been made concerning my employment.

Signature: _____

Date: _____

THE BOTTOM LINE

At-will employees are free to quit at any time for any reason. Likewise, the employer is free to terminate the employment relationship at any time for any reason, unless, of course, the reason for termination is illegal (e.g., violates the Civil Rights Act, ADA, or any other state or federal employment law). At-will employment is governed by state law, meaning that it is the state's decision whether to adopt the standard. Make sure that you know whether at-will employment is applicable in your state.

Rejected applicants

Once you have determined that an applicant does not fit your unit, send the applicant a written notification that he or she was not selected. Doing so is not only courteous but also may prevent any allegations that a job offer was extended to the applicant when in fact no job offer was made.

The best rejection letter is one that is short, simple, and positive. Simply thank the applicant for the interview and let him or her know that another person has been selected for the position. No additional information is necessary, including why the particular applicant was not selected for the position. See Figure 3.4 for a sample rejection letter.

Figure 3.4 Sample Rejection Letter

January 1, 2016

Dear Nurse Martin,

Thank you for taking the time to meet with me last Friday to discuss the nursing positions open at West Lake Hospital. You were among many fine applicants who interviewed for the job. I wanted to let you know that we selected another applicant for the position.

It was a pleasure meeting you, and I wish you well in your job search.

Signature: _____

[insert name], Nurse Manager

Orientation

Once hired, the new employee must complete orientation to the facility and to your unit. In this context, you as the nurse manager must verify that the employee is competent to operate all equipment on the unit, can competently provide care on the unit, and knows the unit's policies and procedures. Make sure to document that the orientation was successfully completed and that the nurse is cleared to practice nursing on your unit. If you fail to complete the nurse's orientation to verify competency on the unit—or if you fail to document it—then as the nurse manager, you may be held legally accountable if the nurse practices below the standard of care and is found liable for professional negligence.

Conclusion

By consistently and effectively completing these five major steps of the hiring process, you will staff your unit with competent nurses which will reduce your legal liabilty risk.

4

The Legal Significance of Policies and Procedures

Nurse Manager Job Description

The nurse manager maintains nursing and unit standards by writing, enforcing, and updating operational policies and procedures.

Learning objectives

After reading this chapter, the participant will be able to do the following:

- List the purposes of policies and procedures
- Define the duty of the nurse manager in enforcing policies and procedures
- Discuss how hospital policies and procedures are applied in court

In addition to the state and federal laws that regulate nursing practice and define the standard of care, hospital policies and procedures also establish legal standards for nursing practice. Hospital policies and procedures are the formalized written principles under which a hospital manages its organization. They define the hospital's philosophy, patient and staff safety expectations, standard of care expectations, and regulatory compliance practices. According to *Policies and Procedures for Healthcare Organizations: A Risk Management Perspective*, policies and procedures fulfill the following important purposes:

1. Facilitate adherence with recognized professional practices

2. Promote compliance with regulations, statutes, and accreditation requirements

3. Reduce practice variation

4. Standardize practices across multiple entities within a single health system

5. Serve as a resource for staff, particularly new personnel

6. Reduce reliance on memory (Irving, 2014)

The Role of Policies and Procedures

In the simplest of terms, hospital policies and procedures answer the question, "How do we do things in this hospital?" Look at your hospital policies and procedures as your compass for consistency. Patients want and expect to be treated in a consistent, professional manner when they are in your hospital, and written policies and procedures ensure that all staff have a compass to follow for providing consistent care.

As the nurse manager, you have two duties regarding the enforcement of policies and procedures. First, you must ensure that all employees are educated regarding the policies and procedures in effect on your unit. As discussed in Chapter 3, this education should occur when the nurse begins employment or any time that the unit's operational policies and procedures change.

Second, as the nurse manager, you must diligently monitor the policies and procedures to ensure that they are current and that they accurately represent the work that your staff completes on a daily basis.

Be mindful that when a clinical procedure changes or a new medical device is introduced on your unit, you should review policies and procedures to make sure that they reflect the new practice. If they do not, you must update the policy to implement the new standard on your unit.

THE BOTTOM LINE

If a policy or procedure changes, each member of your staff must complete and document a competency assessment to ensure that they are practicing within the newly established standards.

Policies and procedures in court

Although hospital policies and procedures are not law, you face significant legal consequences if these internal standards are violated. When a nurse assumes care of a patient, that nurse is expected to operate in accordance with the policies and procedures that have been adopted by his or her employing facility. If a patient is injured while under the nurse's care, one of the first elements that the plaintiff's attorney will investigate is whether the nurse provided care according to the hospital's established policies and procedures. If the nurse did not, then the plaintiff's attorney may be able to show that the nurse's practice was below the standard of care.

As the nurse manager, you must monitor your staff's compliance with your hospital's policies and procedures. If you determine that the nurse is practicing outside established policies and procedures, immediately address the situation with the nurse.

First, reeducate the nurse about the specific policy and procedure, and ensure that the nurse understands what is required under the policy. Then, ask the nurse whether he or she will be able to meet the requirements of the policy and procedure. If necessary, have the nurse demonstrate competency. Document what occurred in this meeting, and maintain the documentation in the nurse's personnel file.

If the nurse continues to violate the policy and procedure, it may be necessary to complete a disciplinary action. Document each discussion you have with the nurse regarding the policy and procedure. Later, if the nurse is sued for having harmed a patient while violating the policy and procedure, you can produce documentation proving that you took appropriate corrective actions, which may reduce your liability.

As the nurse manager, you may be liable if it is documented in the nurse's personnel file that the staff nurse was practicing outside an established policy and procedure and that you failed to either address the situation to ensure that the nurse was competently following the policy and procedure or terminate the employee for noncompliance.

Violation of hospital policies and procedures

Courts generally rule against nurses who violate employers' policies and procedures. For example, in *Beck v. Director, Arkansas Employment Security Department,* 987 S.W.2d 733 (Ark. App., 1999), the court upheld the termination of a nurse who intentionally violated the medication policies and procedures of her institution. In this case, organizational policies and procedures dictated that medications were to be charted when administered to the patient. The nurse stated that she made it her practice to chart all her medications at the end of the shift.

On the day in question, when the nurse went to chart her medications at the end of the day, the nurse admitted that she could not remember what medications she had given or to whom. The nurse also had administered Darvocet without checking the patient's medication orders first; consequently, the patient received the medication earlier than ordered. The nurse was legally terminated for having intentionally violated hospital policies and procedures.

THE BOTTOM LINE

You may be liable if it is documented in a nurse's personnel file that the staff nurse was practicing outside an established policy and procedure and that you failed to address the situation appropriately.

Defining policies and procedures in educational materials

Hospital policies and procedures are the formal written principles that guide an organization, but according to some court decisions, these policies and procedures also may include educational videos or programs, training materials, or certifications that a hospital requires of its employees. This is demonstrated in the following case.

In *Santa Rosa Medical Center v. Robinson,* 560 S.W.2d 751 (Tex. Civ. App., 1977), a patient sustained a head injury and developed permanent brain damage following an altercation with a nursing assistant on a psychiatric unit. The lawsuit alleged, in part, that nursing staff were negligent in failing to notify the patient's physician of the head injury in a timely manner. Evidence introduced at trial included video training materials containing in-depth analysis of head injuries and an instructional guide. These educational materials, which addressed the nature and common symptoms of head injuries, were required training for personnel in the hospital and established a standard under which head injuries were to be evaluated. These training materials established policy and procedure for the hospital and set expectations that the staff were required to follow. When the staff practiced outside these established standards, liability was assigned to the hospital.

Risk of allowing unwritten policies

Courts also have assigned liability for unwritten policies. In *Hartman v. Riverside Methodist Hospital*, 577 N.E.2d 112 (Ohio App., 1989), Mrs. Hartman underwent a surgical procedure after eating a full meal. The post-operative nurses were informed that the patient had received Fentanyl and had eaten a meal. Aspiration precautions were not implemented, and Mrs. Hartman died of aspiration after receiving pain medication.

The attending physician had an unwritten policy that no medication was to be given to his patients without first consulting him and receiving medication orders. The nurse attending Mrs. Hartman was aware that the physician did not want pain medications given to his post-operative patients without his approval and that this was the physician's common practice. In this case, even though there was no written policy, the nurse was found professionally negligent for having violated an unwritten policy.

THE BOTTOM LINE

If you as a nurse manager know that a physician has an unwritten policy regarding how he or she wants patients handled on your unit, make sure to have the physician write a standing order. As the above case indicates, unwritten practices may have legal ramifications; however, unwritten policies may change without notice or may not be recalled correctly when a person is testifying in court. Written policies and procedures are always the best legal defense.

Keeping Staff Education and Certifications Current

Staff education does not end once a nurse completes orientation—it is an ongoing process that must be monitored continually to ensure that all certifications and trainings are current. If certifications and trainings are not current, the plaintiff's attorney can use this information as evidence against the hospital when a patient is injured.

For example, if your unit is sued in a wrongful death action after unsuccessful emergency resuscitation efforts, it can be very damaging to the hospital's defense if the plaintiff's attorney discovers that one of the nurses working the code was not current in cardio-pulmonary resuscitation (CPR). The nurse's out-of-date certification will raise doubts about the emergency resuscitation efforts afforded the patient.

Let's look at how the nurse manager would be questioned in a deposition regarding a staff nurse with an expired CPR card.

Plaintiff's attorney: *For the record, will you please read your hospital's policy and procedure regarding CPR certification?*

Nurse manager: *(Reading) All direct care staff must be certified in cardio-pulmonary resuscitation (CPR). Direct care staff shall not provide patient care with an expired CPR certification.*

Plaintiff's attorney: *Did Nurse Smith have a current CPR certification on the evening of March 3, 2015, when the code was called for my client?*

Nurse manager: *No.*

Plaintiff's attorney: *Is this a violation of your hospital's policies and procedures?*

Nurse manager: *Yes.*

Plaintiff's attorney: *Who is responsible for ensuring that CPR certifications are current on Nurse Smith's unit?*

Nurse manager: *The nurse manager.*

Plaintiff's attorney: *Are you the nurse manager for the unit?*

Nurse manager: *Yes.*

Plaintiff's attorney: *Would you agree with me that you failed to ensure that Nurse Smith had a valid CPR certification on the date in question?*

Nurse manager: *Yes.*

As you can see, the nurse manager admitted that he or she was professionally negligent because it is his or her duty to ensure that all nurses are current on their CPR certifications. In such situations, your defense if very limited because the policy and procedure established the expected practice. If you practice outside the policies and procedures, you will be liable.

Because you need your staff involved in patient care and not sitting in a classroom, keeping staff education up to date is difficult. Nevertheless, the legal ramifications for out-of-date training can be severe, so monitor your staff to make sure that their training and certifications are current.

THE BOTTOM LINE

It is your responsibility as nurse manager to ensure that nursing staff members are practicing in accordance with your facility's policies and procedures. If they are not, it is your duty to remedy the situation as soon as possible.

References

Irving, A.V. (2014). Policies and Procedures for Healthcare Organizations: A Risk Management Perspective. *Patient Safety & Quality Healthcare*. Retrieved from *http://psqh.com/september-october-2014/policies-and-procedures-for-healthcare-organizations-a-risk-management-perspective.*

5

Dealing With Problem Employees

Nurse Manager Job Description

The nurse manager maintains job performance by coaching, counseling, and disciplining employees and by planning, monitoring, and appraising job performance.

Learning objectives

After reading this chapter, the participant will be able to do the following:

- Explain the legal significance of the yearly employee evaluation
- Explain the four steps of progressive discipline
- Implement the termination process in a confidential and respectful manner

Despite your best efforts to hire and orient employees to your unit, there will be times when an employee isn't meeting expectations. In these situations, your job is to either work with the employee to remedy the situation so that the employee may become a productive member of your nursing staff or terminate the employee.

Confronting problem employees can be very stressful. Even when you have extensive documentation that an employee is incompetent or endangers patient safety, the decision to terminate an employee may carry legal risks. Nevertheless, failing to do so jeopardizes patient safety, interferes with staff morale, and increases liability for both you and the hospital.

To avoid liability in a wrongful termination lawsuit, you must be able to show the court that your decision to terminate the employee was based on legitimate, objective, nondiscriminatory data.

Consistent and Fair Disciplinary Actions

In all your disciplinary actions, you must be consistent. You cannot pick and choose which employees to discipline. If you regularly allow some employees to engage in certain behaviors and then fire other employees for the same conduct, you are setting yourself up for a lawsuit alleging discrimination.

For example, if Annette receives a written reprimand for failing to give a dose of insulin, Bob must receive a written reprimand when he fails to administer a dose of insulin. You must be an honest and fair supervisor. In addition to reducing your liability, treating employees equally reinforces your image as an impartial employer and, consequently, increases employee loyalty.

To be honest and fair, first ensure that your employees know the disciplinary policies you enforce on the unit. By approaching employee discipline in an open and consistent manner, your hardworking, competent employees know that they won't be fired on a whim and trust that those employees who are not meeting the accepted standards will be dealt with accordingly. This security will increase the morale of your dependable employees.

THE BOTTOM LINE

When you make your disciplinary policies well known to your staff, your accountability to those policies and procedures becomes even greater. You must consistently follow those policies and procedures; otherwise, you will lose the confidence and support of your nursing staff.

Employee Evaluations

The yearly employee evaluation is a significant line of defense in identifying and addressing competency issues with your nursing staff. When consistently implemented by the nurse manager, a sound evaluation system identifies issues *before* they negatively affect patient care. Most hospitals require that employee evaluations be completed on a yearly basis.

Employee evaluations have significant legal consequences. Plaintiff's attorneys have successfully used these evaluations to establish that hospitals knew that employees were providing patient care in an incompetent or dangerous manner, thereby establishing that the hospital was liable for patient harm.

THE BOTTOM LINE

The best way to stay current on your evaluations is to mark in your calendar which evaluations are due each month and then to pick a week during that month during which you complete all evaluations.

Impact of unaddressed competency issues

In *St. Paul Medical Center v. Cecil*, 842 S.W.2d 808 (Tex. App., 1992), an obstetrical patient presented to the hospital in active labor and was attended by a nurse and resident physician. The patient experienced extensive complications during labor, and the primary care nurse started both internal and external fetal monitoring, which, three hours into admission, showed severe fetal hypoxia. Ultimately, the infant was delivered by cesarean, but extensive brain damage had already occurred.

At trial, the plaintiff's attorney introduced the employee's evaluation to show that the nurse had documented competency issues. The employee evaluation, which had been completed three months earlier, identified that the nurse had difficulty using electronic fetal monitors, was reluctant to seek assistance from her supervisors, and sometimes fell asleep while on duty. No evidence was introduced to identify that these performance issues had been addressed by management.

Here, the nurse employee was not the only nurse at fault. The nurse manager, who was responsible for completing performance evaluations and correcting competency deficiencies, was also responsible for the adverse patient outcome because the competency issues were never appropriately addressed.

By implementing the following steps, nurse managers can increase the effectiveness of their employee evaluations:

1. Continually observe and document performance

2. Prepare and deliver the performance evaluation carefully

3. Follow up when competency issues are identified

THE BOTTOM LINE

The nurse manager must exercise diligence in completing employee performance evaluations and in following up on any identified competency issues.

Continually observe and document performance

An effective employee evaluation tells the entire story by documenting the nurse's performance for a year. This means you must observe and record each nurse's performance throughout the year—not just in the few weeks before the employee's evaluation.

Many types of information offer insight into a nurse's competency level, and you should collect this information in a performance log for each employee you supervise. This performance log should address incident reports, medication errors, nursing documentation, work attendance, and nursing interactions on the unit. It should also contain objective, job-related feedback from the nurse's direct supervisor, such as the charge nurse, who is familiar with the nurse's strengths and weaknesses as an employee. All documentation in the performance log should provide objective, measurable examples of how each nurse performs his or her job. Refer to Figure 5.1 for a sample confidential performance log.

Recognize the bad-attitude employee

An employee with a bad attitude is very destructive to your unit. The bad-attitude employee complains about everything, shows up to work late, doesn't care about job performance, and is disruptive to the unit. It can be difficult to discipline a bad-attitude employee because you can't terminate someone for being rude, lazy, or sloppy. However, the following techniques provide ways that you *can* discipline and terminate the bad-attitude employee:

- Keep the subjective data that they are "rude" out of the conversation.

Figure 5.1 Sample Confidential Performance Log		
Employee name: Nancy Nurse, RN **Employee title:** Staff Nurse		
Date	**Incident**	**Oral reminder/written warning**
4/20/2015	Medication error: Nancy completed an incident report stating that she missed a dose of cardizem for 56-year-old male. Copy of incident report in personnel file. No patient harm occurred.	Informal verbal reminder given.
4/22/2015	Communication breakdown: Nancy took orders via phone from a physician regarding chest x-ray for patient but failed to execute the orders. Chest x-ray not completed on Nancy's shift.	Informal verbal reminder given.
6/03/2015	Medication error: Nancy administered IV antibiotics to the wrong patient. Incident report was completed by the charge nurse. Nancy unaware of the mistake until brought to her attention by the charge nurse. No patient harm occurred.	Written warning given. Copy in Nancy's personnel file. Nancy verbalized understanding of written warning.
6/25/2015	Nancy 15 minutes late to work.	No action taken.

- Instead of telling these employees that they have a bad attitude, you must discipline them for violating hospital policies and procedures or for not practicing within the expected standards of their job description. For example, tell employees who are constantly late that they are violating the job description, which states that each employee will report to work in a timely manner.

- Always speak to these employees in terms of their job description and the hospital policies and procedures and identify (document) how those standards are being violated. Discuss the bad-attitude behavior within their expected performance duties.

Prepare and deliver the performance evaluation carefully

The performance evaluation should mirror the nurse's job description. Prepare each yearly performance evaluation as if it were a legal document. Support your documentation with concrete examples of how the employee performed his or her assigned job throughout the year.

When meeting with an employee to discuss evaluations, always be respectful. Question the employee, and give him or her an opportunity to provide opinions or thoughts. Some possible questions include the following:

- Do you think you met a specific goal?

- What are the obstacles that you have experienced while working on the unit?

- Where do you need to improve?

- Could you have used additional assistance from me?

The evaluation process is meant to be collaborative, and you must give the employee time to respond.

Finally, work with the employee to establish new goals for the coming year.

Follow up when competency issues are identified

If the performance evaluation identifies that a nurse does not possess the skills to operate within the standard of care, you must retrain the employee. After retraining has occurred, evaluate the nurse's job performance to determine whether skill levels have risen to meet acceptable standards. If they have, document this information, and return the employee to his or her duties. If they have not, continue the remediation process established in your employee policies and procedures.

If, after you completed all steps of the remediation process, the employee still cannot meet an objective, accepted standard, then the employee must be removed from patient care. For some positions, this means that the employee must be terminated from employment.

In the unfortunate instance where an employee is sued and you are questioned regarding whether you addressed an identified competency concern, you must have the documentation establishing that you met your duties as the nurse manager and that you verified that the nurse was competent to return to the unit and practice within the standard of care. The individual employee may still be found liable, but you as the nurse manager will have significantly reduced your liability if you can produce that documentation.

THE BOTTOM LINE

When you have identified that an employee has competency issues, your best defense is that you have addressed the issues and have documented improvement or termination in the employee's file.

Progressive Discipline for Employees

At some point in your management career, it will be necessary to address employee issues and request that employees improve their behavior, productivity, or patient care skills. Practicing progressive discipline is the best way to address such issues and encourage improvement.

Progressive discipline is a process of using increasingly severe responses and remediation steps when an employee fails to correct a performance issue. Progressive discipline generally follows the following steps:

1. Verbal warning
2. Written reprimand
3. Suspension
4. Termination

Depending upon the specific infraction, such as the level of patient safety involved, you may not need to move through each step of progressive discipline. An employee's performance may require that he or she be terminated immediately.

Progressive discipline is a strong defense when you face an allegation that you have illegally terminated an employee. In cases where an employee fails to improve and termination is necessary, your record of progressive discipline establishes that you treated the employee fairly and that you based the employee's termination on solid legal ground.

Human resources disciplinary policies

Before you implement progressive discipline, make sure to check with your human resources department to verify that this is the disciplinary chain they follow. Hospital human resources departments have extensive policies and procedures detailing how the facility implements and enforces its disciplinary process. To avoid liability, discipline an employee within the bounds of those policies and procedures.

To ensure that you do so, first review the disciplinary policies of your facility. Once you are familiar with them, make an appointment with the human resources department to conduct an information-gathering interview. Figure 5.2 outlines the components of a human resources department information-gathering interview.

This interview accomplishes two goals. First, it further clarifies your understanding of the disciplinary policies and procedures in your hospital. Second, it introduces you to the people who work in the human resources department of your hospital. You should know these people well, because there will be times when you need their assistance at a moment's notice.

Because you never know how an employee will react to a disciplinary action, you must take steps to protect yourself from potentially aggressive or dangerous behavior.

First, ask your human resources department about how disciplinary actions are handled when there are concerns that an employee might become aggressive. Follow their guidelines closely. When you feel uncomfortable, request that hospital security stand by to assist you. Your safety is key.

Figure 5.2 Human Resources Department Information-Gathering Interview

Make an appointment with your human resources department, and use the following questions to further clarify your understanding of hospital policies and procedures.

1. What types of personnel issues have been identified on my unit in the past two years?

2. How did the management staff address those issues? Were those actions successful?

3. Is progressive discipline—using verbal notice and then written warnings—effective in this organization?

4. How do you want to be notified when personnel issues are identified on my unit?

5. I have reviewed the hospital's policies and procedures concerning employee suspension and termination, and I understand that written authority must be received to suspend or terminate an employee. Will you review the chain of command with me so I know how to obtain that written authority?

6. To your knowledge, are there any pending legal actions concerning personnel issues on my unit?

7. Have there been any employee Americans with Disabilities Act (ADA) claims made against my unit?

THE BOTTOM LINE

Never discipline an employee without notifying another person, such as your supervisor, about where and when you will take action. Don't jeopardize your safety when disciplining employees.

Verbal warning

A *verbal warning* is the first step in the disciplinary process, and it notifies an employee that he or she is not meeting expectations. Such a notice is appropriate when an employee violates a minor policy or procedure that does not jeopardize patient safety. Note that the verbal warning is a disciplinary action, and your behavior should reinforce that. Don't joke with the employee during the conversation; be serious and goal-oriented.

To administer a verbal warning, address the employee's inappropriate behavior in private. Discuss your expectations of the employee, how the employee failed to meet those expectations, and the consequences that the employee will face if the behavior continues. Also, give the employee an opportunity to provide his or her perspective. Question the employee to determine how he or she can improve and what type of assistance you can provide to promote that progress.

During the meeting, you and the employee should develop a target date for improvement or determine any additional training that might be required. Document what was discussed with the employee and the outcome of the meeting, and place a copy of the documentation in the employee's personnel file.

Figure 5.3 provides a sample memo documenting verbal warning.

Figure 5.3 Sample Memo Documenting Verbal Notice

To: Shelley Smith's personnel file

From: Dinah Brothers, nurse manager

Date: June 12, 2015

This morning, Shelley arrived for report at 7:05 a.m. Report is scheduled to start at 6:45 a.m., and Shelley is supposed to be here at that time. After report was finished, I asked Shelley to step into my office.

I informed Shelley that all day-shift nurses are required to be at report at 6:45 a.m. so they are ready to assume patient care when that report is finished. I asked Shelley if she was aware of the policy, and she communicated her knowledge of the rule. I asked her if there was a reason that she was late this morning, and she replied that she "just slept late." I told her to call the unit the next time she is running late, and she agreed to do so.

I reminded Shelley that she is a valuable part of the nursing staff, and that patient care is delayed when she is late. I warned her that the next time she arrived late without calling in she would receive a written reprimand, which could affect her employment evaluation. Shelley verbalized her understanding.

Written reprimand

If after the verbal warning the employee continues to engage in inappropriate behavior or in practices that endanger patient or staff safety, a written reprimand is necessary. The *written reprimand* is a serious disciplinary action that lets the nurse know that his or her behavior must improve or job suspension/termination will be imminent.

Prior to the counseling session, write the reprimand. The written reprimand should include the specific facts of the employee's misconduct, prior disciplinary actions that already addressed this behavior, and the specific behaviors the employee must demonstrate in order to perform at a satisfactory level. Attach any supporting documents, such as a hospital incident report, to the written reprimand.

Once the written reprimand is complete, schedule an appointment to meet with the employee to formulate a plan of improvement.

Meet with the nurse in a private setting to discuss the written reprimand. Proceed through the reprimand step by step, discussing each relevant point. Give the nurse the opportunity to ask questions, and let him or her know that he or she may provide a written response. During the counseling session, work with the employee to formulate a strategy for improvement and verify that the employee understands the performance expectations.

At the conclusion of the counseling session, ask the employee to sign the written reprimand. Tell the nurse that the signature indicates that the information contained in the document was shared with him or her and does not necessarily suggest agreement with the content. Some employees refuse to sign the document. In such a case, ask the employee to write a sentence on the back of the reprimand stating his or her reasons for the refusal to sign the document. If the employee refuses this request as well, don't attempt to force him or her to sign the document. Simply document the employee's refusal to sign directly on the document.

Suspension

When an employee is suspended, he or she is sent off the job for a specific period of time. As you can imagine, suspending an employee is fraught with potential legal consequences for the employer, so do not make the decision to suspend an employee on your own. Consult with your supervisor and your facility's human resources department. Follow the suspension policies and procedures of your facility to limit your liability.

When deciding to suspend an employee, first verify that the behavior warrants suspension. Evaluate with your supervisor and human resources department whether the employee's behavior was addressed sufficiently through less punitive disciplinary actions. If it is determined that suspension is necessary and legally supported, proceed with the action.

Meet with the employee to inform him or her of the suspension. Begin by discussing the reason for and length of the suspension. Refer to prior disciplinary actions, such as the verbal warning and written reprimand, to support your decision to suspend the employee. Inform the employee of how he or she failed to improve work performance. Educate the employee what needs to be done before he or she is permitted to return to work.

In addition, notify the employee of the consequences of failing to improve work performance after suspension. Generally, an employee who engages in the same inappropriate behaviors after returning from a suspension should be terminated. If you suspend an employee to investigate claims leveled against him or her and the investigation could result in the employee's termination while he or she is suspended, make sure that the employee understands that possibility.

Your other employees need to know that the employee will not report for scheduled shifts during the term of the suspension, but do not discuss the details of the employee's suspension or the disciplinary action. You as the nurse manager must maintain the suspended employee's confidentiality; you do not want to be accused of violating the employee's privacy rights.

Termination

Some workers are unable or unwilling to improve their job performance and must be terminated from their positions. Terminating an employee is never easy, even when you know it is best for patient safety, your remaining staff, and the hospital. Once again, when making the decision to terminate an employee, consult with your supervisor and human resources department.

There are generally two types of terminations. In one, you consistently addressed the employee's behavior but, despite your best efforts, the employee continues to perform below expectations. In the other, an employee's conduct is dangerous or illegal, and one occurrence legally justifies firing the employee. Such conduct includes threats or actual violence against staff or patients, use of illegal drugs or alcohol at work, or endangering the health and safety of those in the workplace.

When you learn about dangerous or illegal behaviors, immediately remove the employee from contact with patients and staff. This action protects the safety of others and reduces your liability for patient harm. Do not terminate the employee immediately; rather, suspend the employee under the direction of the human resources department.

Before you terminate, investigate the allegations against the employee to establish that you acted fairly in reaching your decision. Make sure to document the findings from your investigation, and include them in the employee's personnel file. In a wrongful termination lawsuit, your decision to investigate before terminating will limit your liability.

Deciding to Terminate

In each case, follow the same basic steps in reaching your decision:

1. Investigate the incident
2. Read the employee's personnel file
3. Consult with your supervisor and the human resources department
4. Examine your treatment of other workers
5. Document the decision to terminate and how that decision is substantiated

Investigate the incident

Your decision to terminate should be based on objective facts rather than on unsubstantiated allegations. Gather pertinent information that legally supports your decision. Make sure that the evidence supports the termination.

Read the employee's personnel file

Read the employee's personnel file to determine whether you adequately addressed the employee's inappropriate behavior through prior disciplinary actions. The personnel file should contain your documented progression through the steps of the disciplinary action: verbal warning, written reprimand, and suspension, if appropriate. If the personnel file does not contain these documents, reevaluate your decision to terminate. The legally appropriate action might be a written reprimand.

If you are faced with terminating an employee for dangerous or illegal conduct, it's possible that the personnel file contains no prior disciplinary actions. Nevertheless, even if the employee was an excellent nurse up until this incident, conduct that you have verified to be dangerous or illegal gives you legal grounds to terminate the employee.

Consult with your supervisor and human resources

Share the documents contained in the employee's personnel file with your supervisor and human resources department. Discuss how your documentation supports a decision to terminate the employee. Verify that your decision is legitimate, reasonable, and supported. Once again, closely follow your hospital's policies and procedures.

At this point, it may be necessary for your supervisor or human resources to sign off on the termination. Make sure to have these approvals completed before you terminate the employee.

Examine your treatment of other workers

In a wrongful termination suit, the employee may argue that he or she was treated unfairly and that other employees who engage in the same behavior have not been terminated from their positions. Therefore, to limit your liability, be consistent in handling similar offenses. Ask yourself whether the conduct exhibited by this employee is conduct that *always* warrants termination. Perhaps there have been instances in which an employee engaged in the same conduct and was granted a second chance. If that is the case, then you must have a valid, legal reason for terminating one employee while giving another employee a chance to improve.

Document the decision to terminate

Finally, in an internal memorandum that will be maintained in the employee's personnel file, document your decision to terminate the employee. This memo should be short and concise and should describe the objective reasons for which you decided upon termination.

How to Terminate an Employee

Now that you have reached the decision to terminate the employee, you must inform him or her. Termination will not be a surprise if you have been progressively disciplining the employee and communicating clearly that the employee is not meeting performance expectations.

Prepare for the meeting

During the termination meeting, be respectful and sensitive to the employee. Terminated employees who pursue legal action often do so because they were not treated with respect during the termination process.

1.   Plan what you will say. Don't act on instinct or assume that the right words will suddenly come to you during the meeting.

2.   You may want a witness present during the termination meeting. If you do, choose a neutral person from human resources to sit in on the meeting. This second person documents the exchange between you and the employee in case a record of the meeting is needed for future litigation. At the end of the termination meeting, have the witnessing party write a detailed memo recounting the meeting. Never ask a fellow employee to serve as your witnessing party. If a lawsuit results from the termination, you don't want the plaintiff's attorney to identify any transgression on your part for having asked an involved party to be a witness to the termination.

3.   Take specific steps to ensure the employee's privacy. Hold the termination meeting in a conference room away from the nursing unit. Such a location not only provides privacy but is also a place where you can leave the employee to regain composure once the meeting ends.

4.   Be respectful in your words and demeanor during the termination meeting. You have only one goal in mind: terminating the employee. You do not want to hurt, humiliate, or embarrass the employee; to do so only increases your liability risk.

5.   Be mindful of your security. For some employees, it may be necessary to have hospital security on standby to escort them from the building. If a terminated employee makes any threats against you or the hospital, report those behaviors to your supervisor, human resources, and hospital security immediately. At termination, make sure that the terminated employee surrenders his or her identity badge and any other credentials that would provide access to the facility.

The termination meeting

First, announce the termination decision to the employee. Make clear to the employee that a future with your hospital is not an option. Don't use ambiguous language such as "you are being let go." Using the word "terminate" clearly communicates to the employee the exact action being taken.

Next, explain the reasons for termination. Keep it specific, objective, and short. If possible, end the meeting on a positive note by shaking the employee's hand and wishing him or her good luck. Finally, document the outcome of the termination meeting, and place the record in the employee's personnel file.

Depending on your hospital's policies and procedures, the terminated employee may not be allowed to return to the unit to gather their personal belongings. If this is the case, reassure the terminated employee that their personal belongings will be gathered and returned to them. Policies and procedures may also dictate that the terminated employee be escorted out of the hospital by hospital security. If this is the case, make sure that you tell the terminated employee what will occur.

THE BOTTOM LINE

The best way to ensure that you maintain loyal, competent employees is to discipline those who are not. When you identify a problem employee, you must act upon that knowledge immediately.

6

Safety in the Workplace

Nurse Manager Job Description

The nurse manager maintains a safe working environment by writing and implementing policies and procedures that promote safety and by correctly addressing safety concerns.

Learning objectives

After reading this chapter, the participant will be able to do the following:

- Discuss conscientious objection
- Discuss the impact of violence against nurses
- Explain reasons for violence in the workplace

Nursing is a dangerous profession. Every day, nurses are subjected to workplace violence, contagious diseases and bloodborne pathogens, chemical exposures and respiratory hazards, musculoskeletal injuries, and stress, all of which can lead to numerous physical and psychological changes in a nurses' health.

Nurses have a right to be safe at work and cannot effectively care for patients when they are concerned for their own safety and well-being. Therefore, one of the nurse manager's most important roles is ensuring that his or her staff feel safe at work and, when they do not, that they are comfortable addressing their concerns. The nurse manager must always be mindful of nursing staff safety and be an advocate when that safety is at risk.

One way that a nurse manager works to safeguard the nursing staff is to ensure that each nurse is individually responsible for his or her own safe care. This means that each nurse must maintain competence in all aspects of the area in which they work, including knowing how to operate all equipment safely and effectively, knowing the types of harmful pathogens that he or she may face, and knowing how to protect against those pathogens, such as by correctly using personal protective equipment. When you as nurse manager witness an employee violating a safety-related protocol, the violation must be addressed immediately. A nurse cannot be allowed to continue practicing unsafe nursing that may harm the individual nurse, other nurses on the unit, or the nurse's patients.

As the nurse manager, you must educate your staff members about all avenues available within your organization for supporting the nurse's physical and psychological health. Programs such as occupational health and employee assistance are in place to assist nurses, and the nurse manager must encourage employees to access this assistance freely.

Nurse managers also must know the number of hours that nurses are working each week. When nurses are overworked, there is increased likelihood of patient errors and/or nurse injury. Some facilities may limit the number of hours that a nurse may work in a specific period of time, and these standards must be followed closely to promote staff safety.

As with all violations of hospital policies and procedures, when you address safety concerns or take a safety complaint from an employee, make sure that you document that information in the employee's file and complete other paperwork as dictated by your facility's policies and procedures.

Nursing: The Most Dangerous Profession

When considering persons who are injured at work, many dangerous jobs come to mind, including construction workers, fire and law enforcement professionals, and industrial employees. So it is surprising to note that, according to the United States Department of Labor, more healthcare workers sustain work-related injuries and illnesses than do workers in any other industry (OSHA, 2015). Specifically, the U.S. Department of Labor states that in 2010, 653,900 cases of work-related injury or illnesses were reported for healthcare and social assistance workers. What makes this number even more stunning is that it represents 152,000 more cases of injured employees than the next identified industry.

These numbers are staggering and indicate the vigilance that must be given to employee health. They put the nurse manager on notice that safety must be of utmost concern in your facility, because injury is likely to occur.

Most if not all nurse managers supervise nursing assistants, such as aides or orderlies. As a manager, you should be aware of the results of a 2013 U.S. Department of Labor report on musculoskeletal disorders (MSD) for all occupations. According to the report, in 2013, nursing assistants had an extremely high rate of musculoskeletal disorders when compared to the national average: For nursing assistants, the incidence rate of work-related musculoskeletal disorders was 208 injured per 10,000 workers, while the average incidence rate for all occupations was 36 injured per 10,000 workers. Your nursing assistant staff suffers MSDs at almost six times the average workforce rate (Bureau of Labor Statistics, 2014).

These statistics reinforce that all employees must be vigilant when lifting and moving patients and that nurse managers must be especially vigilant about nursing assistant injuries. This information is not given to scare nurse managers but rather to indicate clearly that nursing is a dangerous profession and that safety must be addressed continually.

Rights of the Nurse When Providing Healthcare

Nurses have ethical and legal obligations to provide healthcare to each and every patient to whom they are assigned regardless of the presenting diagnosis. That said, each nurse has an ethical compass and core principles to which they are committed, and a nurse should not be expected to violate those principles when at work. When a nurse encounters a patient care situation that is in direct conflict with his or her ethical principles, that nurse has the right to conscientiously object to caring for that patient.

Conscientious objection occurs when the nurse objects to providing a specific treatment and/or to participating in a certain medical procedure due to the nurse's moral code (Lachman, 2014). Some examples of conscientious objection may include, but are not limited to, certain sexual and reproductive practices or surgeries, or assisted suicide.

Conscientious objection is addressed by the American Nurses Association (ANA) in *Code of Ethics for Nurses with Interpretative Statements*. In the *Code of Ethics*, the ANA states:

> *When a particular treatment, intervention, activity or practice is morally objectionable to the nurse, whether intrinsically so or because it is inappropriate for the specific patient, or where it may jeopardize both patients and nursing practice, the nurse is justified in refusing to participate on moral grounds (ANA, 2001, p. 20).*

When a nurse exercises his or her right to conscientiously object to patient care based upon his or her moral or ethical values, that nurse must be free from retaliation. Note that nurses have taken legal action against hospitals for retaliating against them in these situations.

Conscientious objection on religious grounds

In *Britton v. University of Mississippi* Civil Action No. 3:11-CV-483-DPJ-FKB (S.D. Miss. 2012), Tanya Britton worked as a nurse in the postpartum unit at The University of Mississippi Medical Center. Ms. Britton, a devout Catholic, believed that abortion, contraception, and sterilization were morally wrong. Therefore, Ms. Britton declined to provide contraceptives to patients and to participate in sterilizations. In her lawsuit, Ms. Britton claimed that, due to her religious beliefs, she was reassigned from the day shift to the evening shift and was forced to work a less favorable schedule—which included that she work on Sundays. Ms. Britton alleged that this schedule change was retaliation against her for refusing to administer birth control and participate in sterilizations.

Ultimately, Ms. Britton was terminated from her position and took legal action against the hospital and her nursing supervisors for discrimination.

Applying criteria

Although conscientious objection is available to the nurse to protect his or her moral principles, it is not to be used to shirk nursing duties or to avoid caring for a patient due to self-interest, discrimination, or prejudice (Lachman, 2014). Conscientious objection should not interfere with or obstruct a patient's healthcare in any manner.

In "Conscientious Objection in Nursing: Definition and Criteria for Acceptance," Dr. Vicki D. Lachman outlines a list of criteria to determine whether conscientious objection is acceptable, which you will find in the following table.

Criteria for the acceptance of conscientious objection

1. Providing healthcare would seriously damage the health professional's moral integrity by constituting a serious violation of deeply held conviction.

2. The objection has a plausible moral or religious rationale.

3. The treatment is not considered an essential part of the health professional's work.

4. The burdens to the patient are acceptably small.
    a. The patient's condition is not life-threatening.
    b. Refusal does not lead to the patient not getting the treatment or to unacceptable delay or expenses.
    c. Measures have been taken to reduce the burdens to the patient.

5. The burdens to colleagues and healthcare institutions are acceptably small.

In addition, the claim to conscientious objection is strengthened if:

1. The objection is founded in nursing's own values.

2. The medical procedure is new or of uncertain moral status.

Dr. Lachman's criteria provide an excellent compass for determining when conscientious objection is appropriate.

Before nurses find themselves in a position where they are compelled to conscientiously object, they should independently assess their moral core. Then they should meet with their nurse manager to discuss specific treatments or procedures that would violate that code and to which they are compelled to conscientiously object.

With the recent concerns regarding Ebola, many may wonder whether a nurse has the right to conscientiously object to caring for a patient with a highly contagious disease. Legally, nurses *do not* have the right to refuse care based upon a patient's diagnoses. Therefore, the nurse does not have the right to conscientiously object to caring for a highly contagious patient. However, a nurse has the right to be adequately trained and to have demonstrated proficiency in approaching biohazard situations.

As is stated in the ANA Bill of Rights for Registered Nurses, "Nurses have the right to work in an environment that is safe for themselves and their patients" (ANA, 2015). With the new and recent outbreaks of Ebola in the United States, hospitals will no doubt reexamine their policies and procedures regarding the assignment of care for highly contagious patients to ensure that their staff are safe and that patients receive necessary medical care.

Workplace Violence and Bullying

One of the most disturbing issues facing nurses today is the violence they face in the workplace. Daily, nurses are subjected to aggressive patients and hospital visitors, both those who intentionally wish to harm others and those who do so as a result of compromised mental capacity. Nurses also face violence from coworkers who engage in threatening and abusive behavior in person or on social media. Violence directed toward nurses is disruptive, has a negative impact on patient care, inflicts emotional distress upon the nurse, and costs healthcare facilities millions of dollars yearly (Speroni et al., 2014).

There are many definitions in the literature to define workplace violence. According to the National Institute for Occupational Safety and Health, workplace violence is defined as "violent acts (including physical assaults) directed toward persons at work or on duty" (Centers for Disease Control and Prevention, 2002). For our purposes, workplace violence will be defined as an act that occurs at work, or on social media, that subjects the receiver to any of the following:

- Aggression

- Harassment

- Physical threats or assault

- Emotional harm

These violent acts toward nurses may be perpetrated by patients, hospital visitors, or other hospital staff.

Patient and visitor violence toward nurses

According to the Centers for Disease Control and Prevention (CDC), over the past decade, healthcare workers "have accounted for approximately two-thirds of the non-fatal workplace violence injuries which required days away from work" (CDC, n.d.).

Workplace violence is a complex issue and involves many factors, including the perception that "violence is part of the job" and that nurses are expected to tolerate workplace violence. With this prevailing belief, it is difficult to end violence against nurses, in part because many incidents go unreported. It has been estimated that more than 80% of assaults on registered nurses are unreported (AACN, n.d.).

Although patient and visitor violence toward nurses is most common in the emergency room or in mental health settings, nurses have been subjected to violence in various clinical settings, including medical/surgical units, obstetrical/gynecology units, intensive care, pediatric units, and long-term care settings (Gillespie et al., 2013). This means that no nurse is safe from violence in the workplace, and every nurse must be prepared to face this issue.

This fact was vividly demonstrated late last year when Minnesota police released a video, secured from hospital security tapes, of an out-of-control patient attacking nurses. The patient entered the nurses' station, began striking nurses with an IV pole, and then proceeded to chase the nurses when they attempted to flee the attack. In this attack, eight nurses were injured, one seriously when she sustained a collapsed lung (CBS, 2014). While the video is disturbing and difficult to watch, it is also highly educational and should caution all nurses regarding the possibility of work-related violence.

Increase awareness

The types of violence against nurses and the reasons for that violence vary. Nurses work with people who are in very stressful situations, who are experiencing health crises that disrupt not just the individual's well-being but also the family's stability. This stress may lead to the patient or the family becoming aggressive toward the nurse. It has been stated that, in these stressful situations, some aggression toward the nurse is inevitable (Speroni et al., 2014).

As the nurse manager, you must advocate for the safety of your nursing staff. One of the concerns voiced by nurses is that nursing administration does not respond when violence is perpetrated against nurses. *The Journal of Emergency Nursing* recently published "Nothing Changes, Nobody Cares: Understanding the Experience of Emergency Nurses Physically and Verbally Assaulted While Providing Care." In this study, it was determined that emergency room nurses do not feel supported by administration when a violent act occurs (Wolf et al., 2013).

Many of these emergency room nurses further indicated that, while they felt supported by their immediate supervisors, hospital administration were more concerned with the image of the hospital and the publicity that would result from filing charges against the perpetrator. As a result, taking legal action against the perpetrator was highly discouraged. This finding means that you, the nurse manager, may have an uphill battle when meeting with hospital administration to advocate for the safety of your nurses. Regardless, you must stand your ground and, when your nurses are victims of violence, take all actions necessary to ensure their safety. This may include confronting hospital administration. If an injured nurse does make the decision to file charges against his or her abuser, that nurse must not face retaliation from the hospital.

The same study also identified several factors as precursors of violence in hospitals:

1. High-risk environments, including long wait times for care, crowded facilities, isolated treatment areas, and lack of security personnel

2. Psychiatric patients, including suicidal and homicidal patients

3. High-risk patients, including patients brought into the hospital by police and patients with a history of violence

4. Impaired patients and visitors, including those under the influence of alcohol or drugs (Wolf et al., 2013)

Finally, the study identified that violence occurs due to nurses' "lack of cue recognition." That is, nurses are unaware of or ignore the signs that a person has the propensity for violence. Although there are times when nurses are assaulted without prior cues of violence, many patients give verbal or physical cues that they may become violent. For example, a patient who was aggressive toward paramedics while being transported to the hospital also has the propensity to be aggressive once in the emergency room (Wolf et al., 2013).

As the nurse manager, you must educate nursing staff regarding the cues that indicate that a patient or visitor may become violent toward the nurse.

THE BOTTOM LINE

Preventing workplace violence must be a top priority for the nurse manager, and you must advocate for the safety of your nurses even if doing so places you in conflict with hospital administration.

Nurse-on-nurse bullying and aggression

Bullying and aggression are frequent occurrences between healthcare professionals. Often identified as lateral violence—a term to describe the "physical, verbal, or emotional abuse of an employee" by another employee—such nurse-on-nurse hostility is detrimental to the nursing profession (ASMN, n.d.). Lateral violence and bullying have been documented extensively and are shown to result in negative outcomes for registered nurses, employers, and patients (CAN, 2008).

Bullying and lateral violence significantly disrupt the workplace. Bullying is defined as follows:

> *Offensive abusive, intimidating, malicious, or insulting behavior, or abuse of power conducted by an individual or group against others, which makes the recipient feel upset, threatened, humiliated, or vulnerable, which undermines their self-confidence and which may cause them to suffer stress (Task Force on the Prevention of Workplace Bullying, 2001).*

Bullying is generally associated with the perpetrator being in a higher level of authority, such as a nursing supervisor who bullies a staff nurse. Lateral violence is considered as behavior between employees of the same status, such as staff nurse to staff nurse.

Bullying and lateral violence hinder patient care in many ways. First, when nurses are victims of bullying or lateral violence, they may become so intimidated that they fail to advocate for a patient because they fear that they will be targeted and ridiculed. Therefore, bullying and lateral violence have a direct outcome on patient care and safety. Additionally, nurses who are victims of bullying or lateral violence have increased rates of work absences, impaired performance, and lower work productivity.

Bullying and lateral violence also may occur online, through social media avenues. In such situations, disparaging remarks are made by one nurse about a coworker on social media. As the National Council of State Board of Nursing states, "Online comments by a nurse regarding coworkers, even if posted from home during non-working hours, may constitute lateral violence" (NCSBN, 2011).

Addressing Workplace Violence and Bullying

As the nurse manager, you must have a "no tolerance" policy when confronting workplace violence and bullying on your unit. First, read your hospital's policies and procedures. Most likely those procedures will state that the hospital implements a "no tolerance" policy toward workplace violence and bullying. If so, that policy must be consistently followed, or the hospital is violating its own policies and procedures.

THE BOTTOM LINE

A no-tolerance policy means that automatic punishment is implemented for infractions of a stated rule, with the goal of eliminating the bullying and aggressive behavior.

As you know from Chapter 4, "The Legal Significance of Policies and Procedures," inconsistent adherence to policies may result in liability for the hospital. Let's look at an example.

The article entitled "Nothing Changes, Nobody Cares" contains the following statement from an emergency room nurse about signs posted in the emergency room regarding violence:

> [The signs stated,] "We won't tolerate violence, acting out, threats, or cursing." The sign also stated that if you acted in any of these ways, you were going to be escorted out by security and police.

> [The emergency room nurse stated,] I have yet to see this happen. I finally asked if we were ever going to act on these signs, and I was told that basically they were just put up for show" (Wolf et al., 2013).

As you have learned in this book, a court may hold that this sign, which states the hospital has no tolerance for violence, is the hospital's policy and procedure for handling violent situations. Suppose that a staff nurse was threatened and cursed at by a patient at this hospital. The staff nurse immediately informs her direct supervisor and the supervisor replies, "It happens all the time; just blow it off." The staff nurse then returns to care for the abusive patient, who attacks her and breaks her arm and several ribs.

Does this nurse have a case against the hospital? Yes, because the hospital's policy states that they do not tolerate violence; however, when the nurse reported the violence, the hospital failed to act in accordance with its own policy of escorting the abusive person out of the facility. The hospital failed to protect the nurse. Here, the hospital would be liable.

THE BOTTOM LINE

If a hospital states it has a no-tolerance policy toward violence, the hospital must follow that policy.

Issues in handling allegations

One issue often reported by staff nurses is that they feel supported by their immediate supervisor but do not receive support from hospital administration. This conflict may place you in a difficult position because your staff nurses are requesting protection from workplace violence but your supervisors—hospital administration—are minimizing the issue. Here, your loyalty must be to your staff nurses, and you must advocate for their safety. This will be difficult, and you will most likely face pushback from administration, but you must work to keep your nurses safe.

Every time you address your concerns with hospital administration, document the exchange in your files. You will want this evidence in the event that the hospital is sued for negligence due to failure to keep the nursing staff safe. Your documentation will minimize your individual liability, because the evidence will show that you continually addressed the situation with your supervisors but that your request for additional safety measures were ignored.

When you are confronted with an allegation that bullying or lateral violence has occurred on your unit, your first action is to investigate the claim. Ask questions to gather specific, objective data about the bullying or lateral violence incident. For example, if a staff nurse comes to you and reports that the charge nurse is "being mean and doesn't like me," you must gather more information. "Being mean" doesn't tell you anything; you must identify the exact behaviors.

Ask the staff nurse to tell you specifics, such as "the charge nurse yelled at me in front of patients" or "the charge nurse grabbed medication out of my hand and told me I was an idiot." These are specific behaviors on which you, as the nurse manager, can and should take disciplinary action.

If, after you investigate, you confirm that bullying or lateral violence has occurred on your unit, follow your hospital policies and procedures to address the issue. In some cases, you will be able to implement progressive discipline.

In some instances, certain bullying or lateral violence behaviors—such as one nurse striking another nurse—will require that the offending party be immediately suspended or terminated. Here, you must consult with your human resources department prior to taking action.

➡ For an in-depth look at how to implement progressive discipline and how to suspend or terminate, refer back to Chapter 5, "Dealing With Problem Employees."

Bullying creates a hostile work environment

Those who engage in bullying and lateral violence are responsible for their behaviors and should be held accountable for them. In *Dookeran v. County of Cook,* 920 N.E.2d 633 (Ill. App. Ct. 2009), Dr. Dookeran's medical privileges were not renewed and he was terminated from his position with the hospital for his bullying behavior toward nurses. Dr. Dookeran, a surgeon, had a history of verbally abusing hospital personnel, including yelling at nurses and calling them incompetent. Through his behavior, Dr. Dookeran created a hostile work environment. Here, the hospital took the appropriate action and terminated Dr. Dookeran.

The American Organization of Nurse Executives (AONE) has developed guiding principles and priorities to reduce workplace violence and bullying. According to AONE, these guiding principles are as follows:

1. Recognition that violence can and does happen anywhere
2. Healthy work environments promote positive patient outcomes
3. All aspects of violence (patient, family and lateral) must be addressed
4. A multidisciplinary team, including patients and families, is required to address workplace violence
5. Everyone in the organization is accountable for upholding foundational behavior standards, regardless of position or discipline
6. When members of the healthcare team identify an issue that contributes to violence in the workplace, they have an obligation to address it

7. Intention, commitment, and collaboration of nurses with other healthcare professionals at all levels are needed to create a culture shift.

8. Addressing workplace violence may increase the effectiveness of nursing practice and patient care (AONE, n.d.)

THE BOTTOM LINE

You have a duty to keep your nurses safe. You must take that duty very seriously and react immediately and decisively when workplace violence threatens your nursing staff.

References

AACN. (n.d.) AACN Public Policy Position Statement: Zero Tolerance for Abuse. Retrieved from *www.aacn.org/wd/practice/docs/publicpolicy/zero_tolerance_for_abuse.pdf*.

ANA. (n.d.). American Nurses Association Bill of Rights for Registered Nurses.

AONE. (n.d.). AONE Guiding Principles: Mitigating Violence in the Workplace. Retrieved from *www.aone.org*.

Bureau of Labor Statistics, U.S. Department of Labor. (2014). Survey of Occupational Injuries and Illnesses in cooperation with participating state agencies, Table 18. Retrieved from *www.bls.gov/news.release/osh2.t18.htm* on May 27, 2015.

CDC.gov—Workplace Violence Prevention for Nurses.

Center for American Nurses. (2008). Lateral Violence and Bullying in the Workplace. Retrieved from *http://www.mc.vanderbilt.edu/root/pdfs/nursing/center_lateral_violence_and_bullying_position_statement_from_center_for_american_nurses.pdf*.

Department of Health and Human Services, Centers for Disease Control and Prevention, National Institute for Occupational Safety and Health. (2002). Violence: Occupational hazards in hospitals. Retrieved from *www.cdc.gov/niosh/docs/2002-101/pdfs/2002-101.pdf*

Gillespie, et al. (2013). Stressful Incidents of Physical Violence Against Emergency Nurses. *The Online Journal of Issues in Nursing: A Scholarly Journal of the American Nurses Association.* Vol. 18, No. 1, Manuscript 2.

Healthy Work Environment Advocacy Guide: Workplace Bullying and Lateral Violence Among Nurses. Academy of Medical-Surgical Nurses. Retrieved from *www.asmn.org*.

Lachman, V.D. (2014). Conscientious Objection in Nursing: Definition and Criteria for Acceptance. *MedSurg Nursing, 23*(3).

Minnesota CBS Local (Producer). (2014, November 6). *CBS Minnesota*. Police Release Video of Patient Attacking Nurses with Bar. Retrieved from *www.minnesota.cbslocal.com*.

National Council of State Boards of Nursing. White Paper: A Nurse's Guide to the Use of Social Media. 2011. Chicago, IL. Retrieved from *www.ncsbn.org/Social.Media.pdf*.

Speroni, et al. (2014). Incidence and Cost of Nurse Workplace Violence Perpetrated by Hospital Patients or Patient Visitors. *Journal of Emergency Nursing, 40*(3), 218–228.

Task Force on the Prevention of Workplace Bullying. (2001). Report of the task force on the prevention of workplace bullying: Dignity at work—the challenge of workplace bullying. Dublin: Health and Safety Authority.

United States Department of Labor/OSHA. (n.d.). Safety and Health Topics: Healthcare. Retrieved from *www.osha.gov/SLTC/healthcarefacilities*.

Wolf, L. et al. (2014). Nothing Changes, Nobody Cares: Understanding the Experience of Emergency Nurses Physically or Verbally Assaulted While Providing Care. Retrieved from *www.whistleblower.gov*.

7

The Nurse as Whistleblower

Nurse Manager Job Description

The nurse manager creates an environment that adheres to the standard of care and ethical behavior and responds appropriately to staff concerns.

Learning objectives

After reading this chapter, the participant will be able to do the following:

- Discuss the nurse's legal duty to report illegal and unsafe practices
- Discuss how the nurse manager could contribute to retaliation against employees
- Understand forms of retaliation that a whistleblower may experience

In a perfect world, there would be no situation in which a nurse was forced to become a whistleblower, because the nurse's concerns would be properly addressed by hospital administration. Sadly, that is not the case, and nurses are often forced to make the difficult decision to seek recourse for illegal or unsafe practices outside their employer's boundaries.

A nurse becomes a whistleblower when that nurse shares information that his or her employer is violating federal and/or state laws or the nurse knows that the employer is engaging in practices that place the public or patients at risk. The nurse reports that information to the appropriate authority, thus "blowing the whistle" on his or her employer.

Duty to Report

As part of their professional role, nurses have a legal and ethical duty to report illegal acts and unsafe practices. Often the *legal duty* to report is established in the statutes of state nursing boards. The *ethical duty* to report occurs when a nurse witnesses a practice with which they are extremely uncomfortable; it "doesn't feel right." In these situations, the nurse is guided to report based upon his or her individual moral compass.

When a nurse witnesses reportable behavior, he or she should first notify the immediate supervisor, often the nurse manager. Consistent with the hospital's policies and procedures, the nurse manager should gather appropriate evidence and documentation to substantiate the claim. The nurse manager must then go to the supervisor and move up the chain of command, always consistent with his or her facility's policies and procedures.

Within the bounds of confidentiality, the nurse manager must keep the reporting nurse informed that the complaint is being addressed and that appropriate action is being taken. The reporting nurse needs to know that the complaint is being taken seriously and that, if there is evidence to support the claim, appropriate action will be taken against the offending person or organization. Many times, the nurse manager will be held to such a level of confidentiality that he or she will be prevented from disclosing what is being done to address the complaint; however, the nurse manager must communicate with the reporting nurse that his or her concerns are being addressed.

Nurse managers should never create an environment in which their employees fear retaliation and, as a result, do not report illegal or unsafe practices. This is the concern of many nurses who, despite being protected by state and federal laws, choose not to become whistleblowers (Curtin, 2013).

Certain nurse manager behaviors can contribute to creating an environment in which a nurse becomes fearful of retaliation. Consider this example:

> *Day Shift Nurse Smith approaches her nurse manager. She states that she is concerned that narcotics are being mismanaged and that there is some evidence that some medications are being diverted. Nurse Smith has documented every incidence she has witnessed and provides that to her nurse manager. Her nurse manager listens to the concerns and then tells Nurse Smith, "I think it would be best if you just forget about this and pay attention to your own patients."*

> *Later that day, the nurse manager begins to worry that Nurse Smith may not "forget about it," so the nurse manager decides to make some changes in the work schedule so that Nurse Smith does not work with the alleged offending parties. Nurse Smith is reassigned to the night shift.*

Here, the nurse manager's actions were clearly based on the fact that Nurse Smith came forward and raised safety concerns. Nurse Smith may have a valid complaint for retaliation.

Nurse managers must make assignments, evaluate employees, and handle their administrative duties in a fair and ethical manner. A nurse manager must never reassign a nurse who comes to him or her with safety concerns or treat that nurse any differently than he or she handles any other employee.

THE BOTTOM LINE

When making assignments or preparing evaluations on an individual employee, the nurse manager must be careful that personal feelings and concerns for his or her own professional welfare are not the guiding objectives. Employee assignments and evaluations must be based upon objective—not subjective— data, regardless of how a nurse manager may feel about an employee.

Nurses are more likely to become whistleblowers when they think that their complaints are being ignored or not taken seriously. Nurses reach this conclusion when they make a complaint and are never notified of any action taken as a result, or when they never hear anything back from the nurse manager. As a nurse manager, even when bound by confidentiality, you must communicate with nurses who make formal complaints regarding the status of their complaint. Nurses also may decide to become whistleblowers when they think that their complaint was ignored or was not handled appropriately. This may be a common occurrence, especially when the nurse's employing hospital is the party suspected of engaging in the unsafe or illegal activities.

The decision to become a whistleblower is very complex and should not be taken lightly. This serious decision should only be made after the nurse has exhausted every in-house avenue and has worked through all considerations.

Deciding to become a whistleblower

The American Nurses Association has identified numerous elements to consider when making the decision to become a whistleblower. In *Things to Know About Whistle Blowing* (ANA, n.d.), the ANA holds the following:

- If you identify an illegal or unethical practice, reserve judgment until you have adequate documentation to establish wrongdoing.

- Do not expect those who are engaged in unethical or illegal conduct to welcome your questions or concerns about this practice.

- Seek the counsel of someone you trust outside of the situation to provide you with an objective perspective.

- Consult with your state nurses association or legal counsel if possible before taking action to determine how best to document your concerns.

- Remember, you are not protected from retaliation by your employer in a whistleblower situation until you blow the whistle.

- Blowing the whistle means that you report your concern to the national and/or state agency responsible for regulation of the organization for which you work or, in the case of criminal activity, to law enforcement agencies.

- Private groups, such as The Joint Commission or the National Committee for Quality Assurance, do not confer protection. You must report to a state or national regulator.

- Although not required by every regulatory agency, it is a good rule of thumb to put your complaint in writing.

- Document all interactions related to the whistleblowing situation, and keep copies for your personal file.

- Keep documentation and interactions objective.

- Remain calm and do not lose your temper, even if those who learn of your actions attempt to provoke you.

- Remember that blowing the whistle is a very serious matter. Do not blow the whistle frivolously. Make sure that you have the facts straight before taking action.

This list provides a comprehensive framework for guiding a nurse who is weighing the decision to become a whistleblower.

As the nurse manager, you may find yourself in the position where you yourself are forced to become a whistleblower. In a management position, you will have access to standard of care issues, limited financial information regarding your hospital, and liability and risk issues. This information may alert you to hospital or individual practitioner practices that are illegal or unethical. When this occurs, follow the steps outlined above, and move through the chain of command.

Make sure that you document every step you take in the process so that, if you are retaliated against, you will have the data necessary to take legal action against your employer. If you find yourself in a position where you are compelled to become a whistleblower, consult with an attorney before moving forward.

Whistleblower Retaliation

Retaliation is real and can have a negative impact on the whistleblower. Nurses who make the decision to become whistleblowers may be faced with retaliation from their employers, including but not limited to the following:

- Changes in work assignments or shifts, including increased patient acuity

- Isolation from peers, often because peers are fearful for their own jobs

- Threats from upper management regarding professional and personal reputation

- Reduced opportunities for professional advancement within the organization

- Termination from employment

On a personal level, nurses who make the decision to become whistleblowers may face psychological issues, such as anxiety or depression (Patterson, 2012). Nurses must know that this is possible and have a plan in place regarding where to seek support and how to deal with these psychological issues.

In 2009, two Texas nurses faced extreme retaliation when they decided to report a physician to the Texas Medical Board for practice below the standard of care. The nurses had addressed their concerns with hospital administration but did not believe that the concerns had been adequately handled within their facility. Because they feared retaliation, the two nurses submitted an "anonymous" complaint to the Texas Medical Board alleging that Rolando Arafiles, MD, was practicing medicine below the standard of care. These two nurses, Anne Mitchell, RN, and Vicki Galle, RN, were employed in quality improvement/risk management positions at the hospital where Dr. Arafiles practiced medicine.

Upon learning of the medical board complaint, Dr. Arafiles approached the county sheriff, who was a patient and a friend, and asked the sheriff to help him determine who had made the complaint to the medical board. Dr. Arafiles was able to identify the patients named in the complaint, and he pulled the patients' medical records. Dr. Arafiles then gave that confidential information to the sheriff, who interviewed each of the ten patients to determine whether any of them made the complaint against Dr. Arafiles.

Once he determined that none of the patients had made the complaint, the sheriff (in his official capacity) contacted the medical board and requested a copy of the complaint. The sheriff used the copy of the complaint, along with other information, to identify the two nurses.

Once the identity of the two nurses was known, they were terminated from their positions at the hospital and indicted on criminal charges for misuse of official information (In the Matter of the Complaint Against Rolando German Arafiles, M.D. Texas State Office of Administrative Hearings. SOAH Docket No. 503-10-4941. June 22, 2010.). Following a jury trial, Nurse Mitchell was acquitted, and the charges against Nurse Galle were dropped.

As a result of his actions, Dr. Arafiles pleaded guilty to criminal charges of retaliation and misuse of official information, which is a third-degree felony in Texas (Lower, 2011). Dr. Arafiles voluntarily and permanently surrendered his medical license to the Texas Medical Board for commission of a felony (In the Matter of the Complaint Against Rolando German Arafiles, M.D. Texas State Office of Administrative Hearings. SOAH Docket No. 503-10-4941. Voluntary Surrender Order. Nov. 4, 2011.).

This case and the retaliation against the nurses in question received extensive media coverage, including coverage from the *New York Times*. These two nurses were persecuted for having followed the law and stood up for patient safety. They made the correct decision to stand up for patient safety and welfare.

Federal and State Protection

Many state and federal laws protect whistleblowers from retaliation by their employers. Under federal law, OSHA governs the whistleblower protection provisions. These federal statutes prohibit employers from retaliating or discriminating against an employee for having engaged in whistleblower activity. Persons who have been the victims of retaliation may file a complaint with OSHA (OSHA, n.d.).

State law also protects employees from retaliation. When making the determination to become a whistleblower, consult your state law regarding your protection from retaliation. The best way to do this is to consult with an experienced attorney.

References

ANA. (n.d.). Things to Know About Whistle Blowing. Retrieved from *www.nursingworld.org/MainMenuCategories/ThePracticeofProfessionalNursing/workforce/Workforce-Advocacy/Whistle-Blowing.html.*

Curtin, L.L. (2013). When nurses speak up, they pay a price. *American Nurse Today, 8*(10).

Lower, R. (2011). Texas Physician Pleads Guilty in Whistle-Blowing Nurses Case. Retrieved from *www.medscape.com/viewarticle/753029.*

Patterson, K. (2012). RN whistle-blowers summon moral courage. *Nurse.com.* Retrieved from *http://news.nurse.com/article/20120402/NATIONAL01/104020020.*

Sack, K. (2010, February 11). Whistle-Blowing Nurse Is Acquitted in Texas. *The New York Times.* Retrieved from *http://www.nytimes.com/2010/02/12/us/12nurses.html?_r=0.*

United States Department of Labor, Occupational Safety & Health Administration. The Whistleblower Protection Programs. Retrieved from *www.whistleblowers.gov.*

8

The Liability Risks
of Nurse Staffing

Nurse Manager Job Description

The nurse manager ensures that patient care is provided within the standard of care by scheduling and assigning adequate nursing staff to accommodate patient acuity levels.

Learning objectives

After reading this chapter, the participant will be able to do the following:

- Identify the liability risks associated with inadequate staffing
- Explain the nurse manager's responsibility for agency nurses
- Define patient abandonment in the context of inadequate staffing

As the nurse manager, you will continually face the stress of ensuring that your unit is adequately staffed to deliver patient care. You'll meticulously work to schedule the correct number of legally qualified staff for your patient acuity level and then, at the last minute, you'll be forced to scramble when someone calls in sick. Staffing is stressful and frustrating, but it is also one of the most critical duties you will complete in your daily role as nurse manager.

Research has identified that the nurse-to-patient staffing ratio significantly impacts patient outcomes. In general, when the unit is staffed with fewer registered nurses, patient outcomes and patient safety are compromised. One study, *Hospital Nurse Staffing and Patient Mortality, Nurse Burnout, and Job Dissatisfaction,* found that in hospitals where nurses were assigned to care for more patients, there were higher mortality rates for surgical patients (Aiken et al., 2002). Another study concluded that for every additional patient assigned to a nurse, the rate of infection increased (Cimiotti et al., 2012). Although these are only two examples, there are numerous research findings indicating that when nurses are asked to care for too many patients, patient safety is compromised.

Plaintiffs' attorneys frequently argue that high nurse-to-patient ratios result in substandard nursing care, increased mistakes, and patient injuries. As the research studies above indicate, this argument is valid— patients are being harmed because there are not enough nurses to provide care.

When you identify inadequate staffing on your unit, take immediate steps to remedy the situation. Follow your hospital policies and procedures to secure additional staff either by reassigning personnel or calling in agency nursing staff. You must notify hospital administrators regarding your staffing concerns.

THE BOTTOM LINE

To minimize your liability, make sure to document all your efforts to remedy the staffing issue, including notices you provided to your supervisors regarding your concerns.

Laws Governing Staffing

Although we will not go into great detail on this issue here, be aware that there are both state and federal laws that govern staffing. Federal law mandates that hospitals receiving Medicaid must "have adequate numbers of licensed registered nurses, licensed practical (vocational) nurses, and other personnel to provide nursing care to all patients as needed" (42 *CFR* 482.23(b)).

Some states have enacted state laws that mandate nurse-to-patient staffing ratios or require hospitals to have staffing committees responsible for staffing policies. One resource to identify your state's laws is the American Nurses Association's *Nurse Staffing Plans & Ratios*. If your state enforces staffing laws, you must staff to ensure compliance with those laws.

Is nurse staffing a liability risk?

As early as 1965, courts recognized that hospitals have a duty to provide a sufficient number of staff to continuously monitor a patient's condition (*Darling v. Charleston Memorial Hospital,* Ill. Sup. Ct. 33 Ill 2d. 326, 211 N.E.2d. 253 [1965]). Short (or inadequate) staffing occurs when a unit does not have enough professionally trained personnel to meet patient care needs. When evaluating inadequate staffing, courts analyze this question on a case-by-case basis, depending on a careful, objective analysis of the number of patients on the unit, patient acuity, and the amount of care required by each patient compared to the number and qualifications of staff members on duty.

When nurse staffing is found to be inadequate, hospital management may be held liable for patient injuries that occur as a result of short staffing. This was the issue in a case that directly attributed the death of a patient to a staffing shortage and to the administration's refusal to address the situation. In *Living Center of Texas v. Penalver,* 256 S.W.3d 678 (Tex. 2008), a nursing home resident died after she was dropped while being transferred from her wheelchair to the bed. The resident's care plan called for two people to assist any time the patient was transferred, but the nurse's aide who was assisting the resident was not aware of the information in the care plan. The nurse's aide testified that she had not read the care plan due to lack of time. On the day in question, two nurse's aides called in sick, leaving the facility short-staffed. Although the administrator and the director of nursing knew that the facility was critically short-staffed, they did not arrange for additional personnel.

Here, the nursing home, the administrator, and the nursing director were found liable for the resident's death because they took no action to secure additional staff to provide patient care. This decision is significant for nurse managers, because it indicates that nurse managers who know that an inadequate staffing situation exists must take steps to address the staffing issues, or they will be held liable for patient injuries that occur as a result of that staff shortage. To demonstrate such liability, the plaintiff's attorney must establish that the patient's injury was a direct result of inadequate staffing and was not due to the individual nurse's incompetence.

> **A practical application of the law: Addressing staffing shortages**
>
> When you recognize that your unit is short-staffed, notify your supervisor and/or hospital administrators. You must call in additional staff to secure patient safety.
>
> Assigning staff properly is critical. This means your staff assignments have the correct numbers of registered nurses, licensed vocational (practical) nurses, and nursing support staff. If a registered nurse calls in sick, that registered nurse must be replaced with another registered nurse, not with a nurse's aide.
>
> Often, when units are short-staffed, nurses or nursing support staff attempt to perform duties beyond their current skills and abilities. You must make certain that your nurses understand and practice within their skill limits. As always, document the actions you took to address specific staffing issues.

Intentional short-staffing

At some point in your career, you will be asked to explain your staffing pattern and why it is so expensive to staff your unit. You'll be encouraged to "try to cut back" to reduce your staffing budget. In some hospitals, budgetary reasons guide staffing decisions. When you are confronted with this issue and are encouraged to cut your staff, consider how it will impact patient safety.

Intentional understaffing opens the door to legal liability because, from the minute the shift begins, your nursing staff will be unable to meet the needs of patients. In a California case, intentional understaffing resulted in a $2.2 million verdict (later reduced to $1.27 million due to California's damage-cap statute) because a patient was injured when she fell while going to the bathroom, and the director of nursing, the facility administrator, and the facility owner were found to have intentionally understaffed the night shift (*Saucedo v. Cliff View Terrace,* 2011 WL 680212 [Cal. App., Feb. 28, 2011]).

Be prepared for this inevitable conversation with your supervisor, and know how you are going to handle the request to reduce your staffing. Respond to such a request with factual information, such as, "I know it is expensive to staff the unit, but due to the high acuity of our patients, it would be negligent to reduce our staff." Document this conversation because, if a patient is injured and a lawsuit is filed, this documentation will mitigate your liability for intentional short-staffing because you addressed the issue with your supervisors.

 THE BOTTOM LINE

As the nurse manager, your job is to know the "ins and outs" of your unit, to be very familiar with the acuity level of your patients, and to know the number of qualified staff members needed to care for those patients. If a lawsuit is filed, it will be very difficult for you to defend short-staffing patterns because you—the nurse manager—are expected to be the authority regarding the staffing needs of your unit.

Agency nurses and liability

For many hospitals, agency nurses are used to fill in when inadequate staffing exists. On paper, this may look like the correct action to take—a nurse was needed on the unit, and that nurse was supplied by an agency, thereby meeting staffing requirements. However, using agency nurses is fraught with liability and, as the nurse manager, you must understand that liability.

Nurse staffing agencies enter into a contract with hospitals to provide nursing staff to healthcare facilities. The staffing agency verifies the qualifications of the nurse, including but not limited to appropriate credentials, licenses, and a criminal background check. These agency nurses then report to work on your unit, but they are unfamiliar with the policies and procedures of the unit, where equipment and supplies are stored, and the chain of command. Being unfamiliar with the work setting makes it more likely that errors will occur in patient care.

As the nurse manager, you must view your responsibility for agency nurses the same way that you view your responsibility for the nurses who work full-time on your unit. In fact, numerous court decisions have held the hospital, *not the agency*, responsible when an agency nurse is found liable for professional negligence.

As discussed in Chapter 1, "The Legal Environment of Nursing Management," the legal theory of *respondeat superior* comes into play here. To quickly review, *respondeat superior* is based on the premise that employers are liable for negligent acts of their employees. Hospitals and other healthcare providers are engaged in the business of providing healthcare to the public, and that healthcare facility is responsible for hiring competent, skilled employees to deliver that care. Therefore, when a nurse who is employed by a specific hospital is found to be negligent, the employing hospital may be assigned liability because the nurse's negligent act occurred in the scope of their employment.

When it comes to agency nurses, the question is which entity—the hospital or the staffing agency—had control of the agency nurse at the time that the nurse was negligent. When an agency nurse is working at a hospital, it is generally recognized that the entity that had control of the nurse is the hospital; therefore, the hospital will be liable for the nurse's negligence. Several cases have litigated this issue; we will discuss one of those cases below.

Responsibility for agency nurses

In *Ruelas v. Staff Builders Personnel Services, Inc.,* 18 P.3d 138 (Ariz. App. 2001), agency nurses who had filled in for the hospital on a regular basis abused a patient. The patient sued both the hospital and the nurse staffing agency for the nurses' abuse. The staffing agency argued that the claims against it should be dismissed because the hospital, not the staffing agency, had control of the agency nurses at the time of the negligent act. The Court of Appeals of Arizona agreed and dismissed the staffing agency from the lawsuit. Here, the agency nurses were acting on behalf of another: the hospital. Therefore, the hospital bore the responsibility for the agency nurses' abuse.

This holding has a significant implication for you. As the nurse manager, you are legally responsible for the care provided by agency nurses. You must delegate and supervise these nurses adequately, because failure to do so may result in a professional negligence claim. You are the one who is in control of agency nurses when they are on your unit. You will most likely be asked to evaluate their performance and give feedback to their employing agency regarding that performance. This is additional evidence that you and the hospital—not the agency—are responsible for the agency nurses when they are on your unit. Additionally, if you witness an agency nurse practicing in an unsafe manner, you must immediately remove the agency nurse from patient care just as you would a nurse employed by your facility.

To minimize your liability risk when utilizing agency nurses, implement the following procedures:

1. Identify a group of agency nurses and, when possible, use those people on a recurring basis so that they are more familiar with your hospital's policies and procedures, unit layout, and patient care expectations.

2. Orient agency nurses to your unit. The orientation you provide to agency nurses will be an abbreviated version of what you provide to your staff nurses, but you must provide agency nurses with a standardized orientation before they assume patient care responsibilities.

3. Educate your charge nurses regarding agency nurses, and instruct them to monitor the work of agency nurses closely.

4. Identify the specific responsibilities and duties of the agency nurse. If a particular patient treatment requires specific, detailed skills, assign that task to a full-time nurse who has demonstrated competence for that treatment. Do not assume that the agency nurse will be able to complete the treatment competently.

5. Clearly articulate termination policies of agency nurses to the staffing agency, the agency nurse, and your charge nurses. If you or the charge nurse witness the agency nurse practicing in an unsafe manner, remove the nurse from direct patient care and contact human resources immediately. Make sure that the staffing agency and the agency nurse understand that you will not tolerate unsafe practice on your unit.

You will never be completely free from liability, but implementing these measures can reduce your risks.

 THE BOTTOM LINE

For liability reasons, you must consider agency nurses the same as nurses employed by your hospital.

Nurse Burnout

As a nurse manager, when you have a hole in your schedule and need to fill it quickly, it is common practice to ask your registered nurses to work additional hours or to take on additional shifts. Although this may cover your short-term staffing problem, it may also lead to greater problems down the road when your nursing staff experiences job burnout and dissatisfaction.

Research has indicated that nursing staff burnout significantly impacts the quality of care delivered. In *Nurse Staffing, Burnout, and Health Care-Associated Infection* (Cimiotti et al., 2012), the effect of nurse staffing shortages and burnout was found to contribute to urinary tract and surgical site infections in patients.

The same study found that burnout also leads many nurses to be dissatisfied with their jobs. When nurses were assigned more patients, they expressed higher emotional exhaustion and greater job dissatisfaction. When nurses are dissatisfied with their jobs, they are more likely to seek employment elsewhere, which in turn impacts the nurse manager's ability to staff the unit adequately. Not only do departures due to burnout increase your staffing concerns, they also place the unit at a greater risk for liability.

THE BOTTOM LINE

Occasional overtime is necessary on all nursing units, but you must monitor your staff to ensure that they are not working overtime as a regular practice. If you begin to notice that an otherwise competent and proficient nurse is making medication errors or not completing his or her assignments as expected, look to see whether he or she has been working a significant amount of overtime. The errors may simply be related to fatigue.

Patient Abandonment

Patient abandonment is another legal issue that may result from inadequate staffing. States differ in their definition of patient abandonment, but it generally results when a nurse who has accepted the care of the patient unilaterally terminates the nurse-patient relationship without proper and reasonable notice, even though the patient remains in need of care. Once a nurse has accepted the care of a patient, that nurse has a duty to fulfill the patient assignment or transfer the responsibility of care to another qualified person.

The professional repercussions for patient abandonment are harsh because, in addition to liability issues, nurses face discipline by the state board of nursing, including suspension or revocation of their professional nursing licenses.

In *Husbert v. Commissioner of Education,* 591 N.Y.S. 99 (N.Y., 1992), a nurse was notified by her supervisor that one of the day-shift nurses would be required to work an extra shift due to a staff shortage. According to the hospital's mandatory overtime policy, the nurse with the least seniority was required to stay. The nurse agreed to stay but then left after an hour without informing anyone that she was leaving. Twenty-nine patients, three of them ventilator-dependent, were left without registered nurse supervision. Upon leaving the floor, the nurse informed staff that she was going to see the supervisor and that they could page her if an emergency occurred.

The case was brought before the state board disciplinary panel, who found that the policy was appropriate, the nurse was aware of the policy, and an emergency staffing situation existed on the day in question. The state board disciplinary panel ruled that the nurse had abandoned the patients, and her license was suspended for one year.

Staffing and the Aging Nurse

As discussed earlier, nursing is a dangerous profession that is both physically and emotionally taxing. Nursing as a profession also represents an older workforce, which is more prone to injury. In 2013, the National Council of State Boards of Nursing determined that 55% of employed registered nurses were age 50 or older. Even more significant is that within the next 10 to 15 years, it is estimated that more than 1 million nurses will retire. This number represents about one-third of the current nursing workforce (DHHS, 2013).

The aging workforce presents two specific concerns related to staffing. First, older nurses are more vulnerable to injury than their younger counterparts, a factor that must be addressed when making staffing assignments. Research indicates that, in addition to experiencing the common health challenges of aging, older nurses report chronic pain and excessive tiredness related to their nursing duties (Gabrielle et al., 2008). Older nurses also sustain significant musculoskeletal injuries (Letvak, 2005). These finding indicate that the nurse manager must consider the element of age when making nurse staffing assignments.

The second significant issue is the impact that the retirement of these older nurses will have on the workforce. When these knowledgeable, skilled workers leave nursing, they will be replaced by novice nurses who do not yet have the knowledge and clinical skills of their older counterparts. Older, more experienced nurses have the "intellectual capital … and clinical expertise that serves to improve quality patient outcomes … educate new nurses, and inform the discipline of new clinical problems … that warrant investigation" (Collins-McNeil, 2012). As the nurse manager, you must recognize the benefit of employing older nurses and work to retain these nurses on your unit.

Retaining an aging workforce means addressing the concerns of that workforce. Older nurses have stated that the most important aspects in deciding to stay in nursing are as follows:

1. Recognition and respect
2. Having a voice
3. Receiving ongoing feedback regarding performance (Palumbo, 2009)

These findings are significant, because each aspect represents an area over which the nurse manager has direct control. Although the nurse manager may not be able to control compensation or employee benefits, he or she can certainly show older nurses that their skills and experiences are respected and that they contribute greatly to patient care.

THE BOTTOM LINE

Older nurses are valuable to the care delivered on your unit. As the nurse manager, you must validate and respect the contributions they bring to nursing.

References

Aiken, et al. (2002). Hospital Nurse Staffing and Patient Mortality, Nurse Burnout, and Job Dissatisfaction. *JAMA, 288*(16), 1987–1993.

ANA Nurse Staffing Plans & Ratios. Retrieved from *www.nursingworld.org/MainMenuCategories/Policy-Advocacy/State/Legislative-Age*.

Cimiotti, J.P., Aiken, L., Sloane, D., & Wu, E. (2012) Nurse staffing, burnout, and healthcare-associated infection. *American Journal of Infection Control, 40*(6), 486–490.

Collins-McNeil, J., Sharpe, D., and Benbow, D. (2012). Aging workforce: Retaining valuable nurses. *Nursing Management, 43*(3), 50–54.

Department of Health and Human Services. (2013). The U.S. Nursing Workforce: Trends in Supply and Education. Retrieved from *http://bhpr.hrsa.gov/healthworkforce/supplydemand/nursing/nursingworkforce/*.

Gabrielle, S., Jackson, D., and Mannix, J. (2008). Adjusting to personal and organizational change: Views and experiences of female nurses aged 40–60 years. *Collegian, 15*(3), 85–91.

Letvak, S. (2005). Health and safety of the older registered nurse. *Nursing Outlook, 53*(2), 66–72.

Palumbo, M.V., McIntosh, B., Rambur, B., and Naud, S. (2009). Retaining an Aging Nurse Workforce: Perceptions of Human Resource Practices. *Nursing Economics, 27*(4), 221–227, 232.

9

The Liability Risk of Delegation and Supervision

Nurse Manager Job Description

The nurse manager ensures that patient care needs are met by delegating nursing tasks to competent and qualified nursing staff.

Learning objectives

After reading this chapter, the participant will be able to do the following:

- Define nursing delegation
- Discuss the role of the nurse manager and the charge nurse in delegation
- Enumerate the principles of delegation

One of the most important duties a nurse will ever undertake is delegating a patient care task to another person. The Oklahoma Board of Nursing defines delegation as follows:

> *Entrusting the performance of selected nursing duties to individuals qualified, competent, and legally able to perform such duties (OAC 485:10-1-2).*

When a nurse delegates a patient care task to another, that nurse is doing so with the expectation that the task will be completed legally and within the standard of care. Delegation requires the individual taking over the task to assume responsibility for the outcomes.

In your role as nurse manager, you are responsible for the supervision of various personnel who provide nursing care on your unit. These people include licensed and unlicensed personnel, including registered nurses, licensed vocational/practical nurses, certified nurse aides, and unit secretaries. Each of these professional groups has specific job duties and responsibilities and, as the nurse manager, you must ensure that they are practicing only those duties for which they are licensed or that they are certified to perform. Therefore, when you delegate nursing and non-nursing duties, you must do so in a manner that exercises due diligence to ensure that the persons to whom you are delegating are qualified, licensed, and competent to complete the task.

A large part of your unit's delegation responsibilities rest with your charge nurses. On a shift-by-shift basis, the charge nurse is responsible for delegating tasks to the members of the nursing staff on the shift. As nurse manager, you may find yourself in a difficult position because you aren't directly involved in the daily delegation of nursing and non-nursing tasks, but you may still retain liability if delegation is negligent. In this case, it is imperative that you trust your charge nurses and make clear to them that under no circumstance is an unlicensed person to be assigned duties and responsibilities for which they are unqualified or unlicensed.

You must always reinforce the message that you will not tolerate a charge nurse who delegates tasks beyond the scope of a person's licensing credentials and competency levels.

Delegation and the Charge Nurse

To ensure that the charge nurses on your unit understand your position on delegation, meet with each charge nurse individually. At each meeting, make it clear that you consider delegation one of the most significant responsibilities that the charge nurse will complete. If your state nursing board addresses and defines delegation in its practice act and rules, share that information with the charge nurse. For example, if you are a nurse manager in Oklahoma, share the Oklahoma Board of Nursing's statutes with your charge nurses.

Ask your charge nurses to discuss their thought processes and decision-making when delegating patient care tasks. You want charge nurses to indicate that they look at the task required and consider whether the individual has the appropriate skills and license necessary to complete the assigned task safely and legally.

Legal delegation requires that charge nurses and, by proxy, nurse managers evaluate delegated tasks to determine where the task falls within the scope of practice. When making the decision to delegate, the charge nurse must determine whether the task being delegated is one that only a registered nurse is legally authorized to perform. If so, then only a registered nurse should be assigned that tasks. When a delegated task requires specialized knowledge or complex patient monitoring, these duties should be assigned only to a licensed member of the nursing staff.

Refer to Figure 9.1 for a scope of practice decision tree based on the Texas Board of Nursing decision-making model for scope of practice (Texas BON, n.d.).

Principles of Delegation

In its Joint Statement on Delegation, the American Nurses Association and the National Council of State Boards of Nursing identified important principles of delegation:

1. The RN takes responsibility and accountability for the provision of nursing practice.
2. The RN directs care and determines the appropriate utilization of any assistant involved in providing direct patient care.
3. The RN may delegate components of care but does not delegate the nursing process itself. The practice-pervasive functions of assessment, planning, evaluation, and nursing judgment cannot be delegated.
4. The decision of whether to delegate or assign is based upon the RN's judgment concerning the condition of the patient, the competence of all members of the nursing team, and the degree of supervision that will be required if the task is delegated.

Figure 9.1 Scope of Practice Decision Tree

Is the act consistent with your state nursing practice act? Do the state's rules or position statement address this specific act?

- If yes, continue.
- If no, STOP. The act is not within your scope of practice.

yes →

Is the activity authorized by a valid order when necessary and in accordance with current policies and procedures?

- If yes, continue.
- If no, STOP. The act is not within your scope of practice.

↓ yes

Is the act supported by positive and conclusive data from nursing literature, nursing research, and/or research from a health-related field?

- If yes, continue.
- If no, STOP. The act is not within your scope of practice.

yes → (to left)

Do you personally possess current clinical competence to perform the task safely?

- If yes, continue.
- If no, STOP. The act is not within your scope of practice.

↓ yes

Is the performance of the act within the accepted "standard of care" that would be provided in similar circumstances by reasonable and prudent nurses who have similar training and experience?

- If yes, continue.
- If no, STOP. The act is not within your scope of practice.

yes →

Are you prepared to accept the consequences of your actions?

- If no, STOP.
- If yes, then:

Perform the act, based upon valid order when necessary and in accordance with appropriately established and current policies and procedures. Assume accountability for provision of care.

5. The RN delegates only those tasks that she or he believes the other healthcare worker has the knowledge and skill to perform, taking into consideration training, cultural competence, experience, and facility/agency policies and procedures.

6. The RN individualizes communication regarding the delegation to the nursing assistive personnel and to the client situation, and the communication should be clear, concise, correct, and complete. The RN verifies comprehension with the nursing assistive personnel and verifies that the assistant accepts the delegation and the responsibility that accompanies it.

7. Communication must be a two-way process. Nursing assistive personnel should have the opportunity to ask questions and to ask for clarification of expectations.

8. The RN uses critical thinking and professional judgment when following the Five Rights of Delegation to be sure that what is being delegated or assigned is as follows:

    1. The right task

    2. Under the right circumstances

    3. To the right person

    4. With the right directions and communication

    5. Under the right supervision and evaluation (ANA and NCSBN, n.d.)

The significance of these principles remains consistent: The RN is responsible for ensuring that delegation is legal and within the standard of care.

Negligent delegation and liability

Negligent delegation has resulted in legal action. *Travaglini v. Ingalls Health System*, 396 Ill. App. 3d 387 (2009), provides excellent insight into negligent delegation and the fact that delegation decisions must be made on a case-by-case basis.

Mr. Travaglini, an 84-year-old man, was admitted to the hospital for observation because he did not feel well. Mr. Travaglini's admitting physician had cared for him for many years and was very familiar with Mr. Travaglini's medical history and current condition. On admission, the physician told the admitting nurse that Mr. Travaglini had difficulty swallowing his food and that he should be assisted and monitored while eating.

Testimony at the trial established that after Mr. Travaglini was admitted, an aide entered his room, gave Mr. Travaglini a sandwich, and left the room. No one from the nursing staff remained in the room to monitor Mr. Travaglini while he ate. Mr. Travaglini choked on the sandwich and died.

The Travaglini family offered expert testimony from a registered nurse, Pamela A. Collins, RN, MSN, who testified to the standard of care. Nurse Collins was well qualified to provide expert testimony;

she had many years of experience as an administrative supervisor and nurse manager on a medical-surgical unit. Nurse Collins testified that, for a patient such as Mr. Travaglini who had a known history of swallowing difficulty that was communicated to the nursing staff, the role of the nurse would be to supervise and manage the care of the patient. Specifically, Nurse Collins testified that it was the nurse's duty to only delegate the task of feeding and monitoring the patient after assessing the experience level of the aide and determining whether the aide was qualified to perform such a task. In this case, the nurse had delegated to the aide without determining whether the aide was qualified to safely monitor Mr. Travaglini while he ate. This was a clear deviation from the standard of care. In this specific situation, the nurse, not the aide, should have monitored Mr. Travaglini's care.

As you may remember from Chapter 1, "The Legal Environment of Nursing Management," Nurse Collins testified to what a reasonably prudent nurse would do in a similar situation. Here, a reasonably prudent nurse would have considered Mr. Travaglini's medical history and would have assumed the responsibility of managing his care. Failure to do so violated the standard of care.

THE BOTTOM LINE

All delegation decisions must be based on this singular question: Is the person to whom I am delegating this task competent, qualified, and licensed to legally perform the task? If not, delegation to that person is below the standard of care.

References

ANA and NCSBN. (n.d.). Joint Statement on Delegation: American Nurses Association (ANA) and the National Council of State Boards of Nursing (NCSBN). Retrieved from *www.ncsbn.org/Delegation_joint_statement_NCSBN-ANA.pdf*.

Texas Bureau of Nursing. (n.d.). Six-Step Decision-Making Model for Determining Nursing Scope of Practice. Retrieved from *www.bon.texas.gov/pdfs/publication_pdfs/dectree.pdf*.

10

The Liability
of Social Media Misuse

Nurse Manager Job Description

The nurse manager will ensure patient confidentiality by educating, monitoring, and enforcing the social media policy.

Learning objectives

After reading this chapter, the participant will be able to do the following:

- Discuss the expectation of privacy in regard to social media
- Enumerate examples of social media misuse
- Discuss the "no tolerance" policy of social media misuse

Social media has significantly changed the way in which we communicate with one another. We are no longer confined to communicating with a small group of friends in our immediate circle; through social media, we are able to share information about our personal and professional lives with the world.

Although social media is a powerful platform for communication, it also raises numerous ethical and legal issues regarding the confidentiality and ownership of the information posted. These ethical and legal issues have a special significance in the healthcare arena, where patients have an expectation of privacy regarding their personal and health information and their photographs.

Nursing is a stressful profession, and one way to deal with that stress is to vent, share, and seek advice and support from other nurses. This is understandable, because we all need support in the workplace. Often nurses seek that support on social media, discussing their workday experiences and posting photographs. However, sharing confidential patient and hospital information on social media is not appropriate and may lead to nursing board investigations and result in civil or criminal charges.

Your duty as nurse manager is to monitor the social media use of your employees. First, you must know and understand your institution's social media policy, and then you must make sure that all your employees know and understand the policy. You must constantly reinforce that policy and educate employees regarding the consequences of violating it. When your institution's social medial policy is violated, the nurse manager must discipline the employee appropriately.

Social media has changed the communication landscape, and all institutions must address how related issues will be handled in their facility.

Definition of Social Media

The scope of social media is broad, but for our purposes, we define it as encompassing, but not limited to, the following:

- Networking sites such as Facebook or LinkedIn

- Personal or professional blogs or online message boards, such as Twitter

- Video- and photo-sharing on sites, such as Instagram and YouTube

A good rule of thumb in determining whether a platform is considered social media is that if it allows you to post information or other content on the Internet, it is considered social media, and therefore it is subject to scrutiny regarding the violation of patient confidentiality.

Researchers define social media as "a group of Internet-based applications ... that allow the creation and exchange of user-generated content" (Kaplan & Haenlein, 2010, p. 61). Again, the key to identifying social media is that it contains content that is generated by an individual or organization and that is then posted on the Internet.

For our purposes, social media is written or photographic content that a nurse posts on an Internet site such as Facebook.

No expectation of privacy

Although there is an expectation of patient privacy in a hospital, there is no expectation of personal privacy when one is using social media. As was held in *Romano v. Steelcase Inc.,* 2010 NY Slip Op 20388, 30 Misc. 3d 426 (N.Y. Sup. Ct., 2010), persons who use Facebook or Myspace accounts do not have a reasonable expectation of privacy.

In *Romano,* the plaintiff filed suit against Steelcase, citing that she had been injured to the point that she had lost her enjoyment for life and that she was confined to her home. However, Romano's Facebook post showed her traveling, having fun, and generally enjoying life. Romano's Facebook page established the exact opposite of what she was claiming in the lawsuit against Steelcase.

In court, Romano attempted to block Steelcase from accessing her Facebook posts, but the New York Supreme Court found the following:

> *When plaintiff created her Facebook and Myspace accounts, she consented to the fact that her personal information would be shared with others, notwithstanding her privacy settings. Indeed, that is the very nature and purpose of these social networking sites, else they would cease to exist.*

> *Since plaintiff knew that her information may become publicly available, she cannot now claim that she had a reasonable expectation of privacy (Romano at 434).*

Here, it must be understood that when a nurse posts on any social media site, even to a small group of private friends, that nurse has no expectation of privacy, and what is posted on a personal social media site may be used against the nurse if a lawsuit is filed.

Additionally, that nurse has no control over where the original post will terminate. The nurse might post to three friends and consider that to be the extent of the post's distribution. However, that post to three friends has the potential to go viral if one of them choses to post it elsewhere, to be seen by thousands of people throughout the world. If that post contains sensitive material, it violates patient confidentiality, exposing the nurse to potential disciplinary action by his or her employer and state nursing board, and inviting civil and/or criminal prosecution. The nurse must always assume that anything posted to a social media site is available for the world to see and, once posted, the material is permanently available even if the nurse deletes it from his or her account on that site.

THE BOTTOM LINE

No information or comment should be made on social media that a person would not personally share with the world or be prepared to defend in court.

Examples of Social Media Misuse

One of the most sacred platforms of nursing care is that the patient has an expectation of privacy and can trust the nurse with their most private personal and medical information. Therefore, the primary concern regarding nurses sharing information on social media is determining whether the information violates patient privacy and confidentiality.

Social media misuse occurs when a nurse shares information about a patient that discloses the identity of the patient or provides information that could disclose the identity of the patient. Additionally, social media misuse occurs when nurses post information that could paint their employers in a negative light or reflect poorly on their employing institutions.

Most nurses do not intend to violate patient confidentiality when posting on a social media site. However, during a social media post, the nurse may inadvertently breach patient confidentiality by disclosing identifiable information about the patient, including physical characteristics, diagnosis, or even the patient's room location within the hospital. The nurse does not have to use the patient's name to violate that patient's confidentiality: If someone could potentially identify the patient based on a physical description or medical diagnosis posted on social media, then that information should not be posted on social media or disclosed in any situation.

The following are cases where nurses have been terminated by their employers, and/or disciplined by their state nursing board, for having inadvertently violated patient confidentiality on social media.

Case 1: Best intentions

A nursing student was completing a pediatrics rotation as part of her nursing education. The student, who had always wanted to be a pediatric nurse, asked a three-year-old leukemia patient if she could take his picture while his mother was out of the room. Of course the child consented, and later that evening, the nursing student posted the picture of the child on Facebook, with comments regarding how much she admired the child's courage and how lucky she was to care for such a brave patient.

In the Facebook post, the nursing student identified the child by his first name, stated that he was receiving chemotherapy, disclosed the patient's age, and included the patient's hospital room number in the photograph—all clearly breaches of the patient's confidentiality. The nursing education program was notified of the breach of confidentiality and, following a hearing, the student nurse was expelled from the nursing program (NCSBN, 2011).

Here, the student nurse had no intention of violating the patient's confidentiality, and she had no malicious intent in posting about the patient on Facebook. If anything, the student nurse was attempting to recognize the three-year-old patient as a brave cancer patient who stayed happy and was doing well. However, the purpose of her post is irrelevant, because the patient's confidentiality was violated.

The student nurse's actions also opened up a potential Health Insurance Portability and Accountability Act (HIPAA) violation for the hospital and exposed the hospital to a possible lawsuit from the patient's family (NCSBN, 2011).

Steps to take

As nurse manager, you must address several elements in this scenario:

1. Your institution's social media policies must address the behavior expected of nonemployees who access your institution for official purposes

2. Before nursing students enter your facility for clinical education, hospital administration must address social media use with the educating institution

3. Additionally, as a nurse manager, you must address your social media policy when you meet with student nurses to orient them to your facility

During nursing student orientation, this case will serve as a perfect example of the consequences of social media misuse. Student nurses must know that they are being held to your institution's policies regarding social media use and the consequences for misuse.

Case 2: Poor choice of words

A complaint was filed with a State Board of Nursing regarding a small-town nurse who wrote blog entries in the online chat room of a local newspaper. In the blog, the nurse referred to one of her patients as her "little handicapper." Even though the nurse did not provide personal information about the patient or identify the patient in any way, her actions could have resulted in the identity of the patient being revealed (NCSBN, 2011).

Here, as above, the nurse did not show any malicious intent in posting about the patient. However, if people in the small town knew the nurse and her patients, it would be relatively easy to determine the identity of the patient, which would result in a breach of the patient's confidentiality.

The nurse in this situation received a warning letter from her state board. The letter cautioned her that further breaches of patient confidentiality would result in disciplinary action (NCSBN, 2011).

Case 3: Inappropriate photograph turns to concerns of sexual exploitation

A nurse at a long-term care facility was sent an email with a photograph of an elderly female dressed in a hospital gown. The photograph showed a female patient bending over and exposing her backside. Based upon the context of the photograph, the image appeared to have been taken inside the long-term care facility in which the nurse worked; however, the identity of the person who sent the email and the identity of the patient was unknown (NCSBN, 2011).

In an attempt to learn more about who had generated the photograph, the nurse who initially received the email sent it to other staff members via their computers and cell phones, in essence "publishing" the email to others. The reactions of the staff members who received the email varied from being concerned about its content to laughing and taking bets regarding the identity of the unidentified patient. Additionally, another staff member posted the photograph of the female patient's backside on her blog.

Even though the photograph was discussed among the staff, no staff member brought it to the attention of the supervisor of the long-term care facility. When the supervisor learned of the photograph, there was great concern for the patient's rights, and an investigation was initiated. Local media also became aware of the photograph, and local law enforcement was notified to investigate potential sexual exploitation of the patient.

After an investigation, the county prosecutor decided not to file charges, but several staff members were placed on administrative leave while the investigation was pending (NCSBN, 2011).

Steps to take

This scenario presents several areas of concern for the nurse manager. The nurse who initially received the email had a duty to notify his or her supervisor immediately and to refrain from forwarding the email to other staff members. Additionally, when other staff members received the forwarded email, they failed to report the incident to the manager. This behavior indicates that the staff, as a group, disregarded their professional responsibilities to the patient.

To avoid similar situations on your unit, you must do the following:

1. Clearly communicate to staff that any situation with the potential to violate patient confidentiality or be embarrassing to a patient must be reported immediately to the nurse manager
2. Reinforce that this information must be shared with other staff members

Case 4: ER photograph

It was widely reported in the media that a New York City emergency room nurse was terminated from her job when she posted a photograph on Instagram showing a trauma room after a significant trauma situation. No patient appeared in the photograph, but the trauma room was littered with the remnants of the medical equipment that had been used in an attempt to save a patient's life. The photograph revealed a trauma room that appeared to be chaotic and in a state of disarray.

The hospital terminated the nurse for having posted the photograph (ABC News, 2014).

Steps to take

Here, the issue is the duty to protect your employer and refrain from posting photographs and comments on social media that may potentially embarrass your employer. The issue with posting photographs on social media, such as the one posted by the New York City nurse, concerns the context of the photograph: Nurses look at the photograph and understand that it indicates the aftermath of a normal emergency room dealing with a significant trauma situation. However, the general public does not understand this. To the general public, the photograph identifies a facility that is in disarray and could indicate that the facility is inadequate.

Understanding the context of what is posted on social media significantly impacts what is appropriate to post. A nurse who is familiar and comfortable with such images would not react negatively to such a photograph; however, the general public, which has no medical exposure, will react negatively. When posting on social media, it is important to understand that those viewing our images and reading our posts do not have the same experiences or background and will interpret information differently.

Malicious Use of Social Media

The majority of cases in which social media is misused are completely unintentional, but social media has on occasion been used to intentionally mock or make fun of patients or their sensitive medical diagnoses. This was the case in Indiana, where a VA hospital administrator (a licensed social worker) was suspended after sending an email containing a picture of a toy Christmas elf posing as a patient, pleading for tranquilizers and attempting to hang himself with an electric cord (US News & World Report, 2015).

This type of social media post is especially egregious because it mocks and ridicules the exact conditions that we, as healthcare professionals, are asking the patient to entrust to us so that we may help. This administrator's act also illustrates that managers are not immune to inappropriate posting on social media. As a manager, you must always be mindful of your own social media use.

THE BOTTOM LINE

When a social media post is malicious or attempts to intentionally hurt or embarrass a patient, immediate suspension is appropriate. Meet with your human resources department to investigate the social media post. Once the evidence establishes that the social media post was intentional and malicious, termination of the employee is appropriate.

Consequences of Social Media Misuse

As seen in the examples above, social media misuse often occurs after a nurse has finished a shift in the hospital and is in the privacy of his or her home, using a personal computer and posting on a personal social media page. Even though the nurse owns the computer and is at home, the duty to protect patient confidentiality does not end when the nurse leaves the grounds of the hospital. The nurse carries the duty of patient confidentiality at all times. This can be confusing and frustrating for many nurses who believe that what they say when they aren't working does not concern their employer.

There are numerous consequences when nurses misuse social media. First, the nurse-patient relationship is destroyed. Violating patient trust may impact a patient's decision to access healthcare in the future or how much confidential information he or she shares with healthcare providers. Additionally, the nurse may be terminated from employment and be subjected to disciplinary action by the state board of nursing.

State nursing boards have many avenues for disciplining nurses who are found liable for having misused social media. Depending upon the statutes and rules of the state nursing board, nurses who misuse social media may be disciplined for the following:

- Unprofessional or unethical conduct

- Moral turpitude

- Breach of confidentiality

- Revealing privileged information

THE BOTTOM LINE

With the predominance of social media, state nursing boards will be forced to examine how they discipline nurses who misuse social media and will most likely adopt new rules to discipline nurses who misuse the Internet and violate patient confidentiality.

Disciplinary actions

Disciplinary actions taken by state nursing boards vary based on the rules and statutes of that state, but any such disciplinary action against a nurse may have a long-term detrimental effect on the nurse's career and future employment opportunities.

In addition to being disciplined by state nursing boards, nurses who misuse social media may also face civil and/or criminal charges. A nurse may be charged with defamation, invasion of privacy, and/or harassment. This was the case with an Oregon nursing assistant, who was arrested after posting photographs of an elderly patient residing at the nursing and rehabilitation center where she worked. The photographs, which she posted on Facebook, showed an elderly patient, nude and incontinent; the nursing assistant also posted derogatory comments about the patient. Following a jury trial, the nurse was convicted of misdemeanor invasion of privacy and served eight days in jail. She was also sentenced to two years of probation plus community service (Wilson, 2012).

In addition to her jail sentence, the nursing assistant was terminated from her position. The nursing assistant voluntarily surrendered her nursing assistant certificate to the Oregon Board of Nursing for "failure to respect client rights and dignity and violating client privacy" (Oregon Board of Nursing, 2012).

Social media misuse may also lead to allegations that federal law has been violated, such as that the HIPAA has been violated. HIPAA is a many-faceted law, but, under HIPAA, healthcare information is private. Therefore, when social media is misused in a way that shares confidential patient information, possible HIPAA violations may occur.

Policies to Address Social Media Use at Work and Home

Policies to address social media use must be clear, must be written in behavioral terms, and must cover what is expected of the nurse both at work and at home. Policies must define what the hospital considers to be the misuse of social media, as well as the disciplinary actions that nurses will face if they misuse social media.

The best policy for a facility to implement is a "no tolerance" policy regarding the misuse of social media. A no tolerance policy states that any misuse of social media, as defined by the employing institution, will be grounds for immediate suspension and termination once the allegations have been substantiated.

Social media misuse

The institution must clearly identify what it considers to be the misuse of social media, such as in the following description:

> *Social media misuse is any content posted to the Internet by an employee of this facility, either written and/or photographs, that identifies a patient or has the potential to identify a patient and violate the patient's confidentiality. Social media misuse also includes, but is not limited to, making disparaging remarks about and/or posting photographs of patients, employers, or coworkers.*

Polices should clearly state that *any information* posted on social media that has the potential to identify a patient will be considered a violation of patient confidentiality. This information includes, but is not limited to, physical descriptions and/or characteristics, medical diagnoses, the location of the patient, any medical treatment/test that was performed on the patient, or information about the patient's family.

Photographs

Policies should clearly state that photographs of patients are strictly forbidden under any circumstances. A patient may not have the legal authority to consent to a photograph of themselves, either due to age or mental capacity. Additionally, a patient may verbally consent to a photograph while in the hospital and later claim that he or she was not able to give consent due to a medical condition.

Knowledge of social media misuse

The policy must also state that any nurse who becomes aware that the hospital's social media policy has been violated shall notify their supervisor immediately. The policy must include that failure to notify the nurse manager of social media misuse will result in disciplinary action.

Education and acknowledgment of social media policy

All employees must be educated about the facility's social media policy and the consequences for failing to comply with the policy. Each employee should sign a statement indicating that he or she has been educated about the policy, understands the policy, and intends to abide by the policy. If your facility implements a "no tolerance" social media policy, your employees must understand it and know that the policy will be strictly enforced. Make sure to include the no tolerance policy within the document that you require each employee to sign.

At each yearly evaluation, employees should be reeducated about the social media policy. All employees must again sign a document indicating their understanding of and intent to comply with the facility's social media policy. The signed document then becomes part of the employee's permanent record. If an employee is then terminated for social media misuse and attempts to fight the termination through the legal system, you will have this signed document that clearly indicates that the employee was educated about the policy and fully understood the consequences of violating any aspect of it.

The hospital's social media policies and procedures may also be used against a nurse who has been educated about and agreed in writing to abide by the policy but who violates it anyway. When a nurse knows the policy yet chooses to violate it, the nurse's misuse of social media may be considered an *intentional act,* which may result in additional legal problems for the nurse.

Professional liability insurance companies may *deny coverage* to a nurse who is sued for social media misuse, especially if the nurse agreed to operate under the hospital's social media policy and then intentionally violated it. Social media misuse in this case is considered even more egregious.

➡ For in depth information about the legal significance of policies and procedures, refer back to Chapter 4.

Nurses who are found liable for social media misuse, either by their nursing boards or in civil or criminal actions, may be reported to national databank registries, which will affect his or her ability to obtain employment nationwide.

THE BOTTOM LINE

Your nurses must fully understand that social media misuse will damage the nurse's personal and professional reputation for many years to come.

Communicating with patients through social media

Establishing and maintaining professional boundaries with patients also applies to social media. Nurses must be diligent about not violating those boundaries by contacting a patient through a social media site. Such contact has the potential to violate the patient's confidentiality.

For example, if a nurse who cared for a hospitalized patient "friends" that patient and then inquires on Facebook how the patient is feeling and whether he or she is doing better since getting out of the hospital, the nurse has violated the patient's confidentiality even though the inpatient nurse-patient relationship no longer exists. As a nurse, you began your relationship with that person in the professional capacity as a nurse, and that professional relationship continues on social media.

Patient confidentiality in small towns or rural settings is even more difficult. Many times, a small town nurse will have a personal relationship with a person before that person becomes the nurse's patient. In such situations, nurses must be especially careful about what they post on social media. It is common for people from small towns or rural areas to be social media "friends" with the majority of people in their community. Some small towns or rural communities may even establish a "newspaper" on social media where community information is posted. Nurses connected to these types of social media networks must be especially conscientious about confidentiality.

Here, the best practice is for the nurse to refrain from posting anything about their work on social media. Although this may feel highly restrictive, it is the only way to ensure that patient confidentiality is not violated.

Accessing computers at work

As nurses in the electronic age, we use computers to perform our daily nursing roles, and nurses must work to safeguard the confidential information contained on those computers. Every employee accessing information, such as a patient's medical records, must access that information only for medically necessary and care-related reasons. If a nurse is not involved in the care of the patient, there is no medical reason to access a patient's confidential data, and he or she must refrain from doing so.

This was one of the issues in a lawsuit filed in Cook County, Illinois, by Elena Chernyakova, seeking $1.5 million in damages for invasion of privacy. Chernyakova, a 22-year-old aspiring actress, was admitted to Northwestern Memorial Hospital for extreme intoxication, where she remained unconscious for close to 12 hours.

Dr. Vinaya Puppala, who was an acquaintance of Chernyakova's but was not involved in her medical care, accessed Chernyakova's medical records. Dr. Puppala also went to Chernyakova's hospital room and photographed her, posting those photographs, along with commentary, on his Instagram and Facebook accounts. Chernyakova's complaint alleges that she never agreed to be photographed and, due to her medical condition, could not have given legal consent. Northwestern Memorial Hospital was quick to distance itself from Dr. Puppala, releasing a statement that Dr. Puppala acted "entirely on his own" when posting about Chernyakova on social media (ABC News, 2013).

In addition to Dr. Puppala accessing the patient's confidential information, even though he was not involved in her care, this case illustrates a number of other issues that we have discussed in this chapter:

1. **No consent:** The patient, due to her medical condition, did not have the capacity to consent to photographs.

2. **Intentional acts:** The posts on Instagram and Facebook were intentional.

3. **Meant to harm or embarrass:** The content of the posts make it easy to argue that Dr. Puppala's actions were intentional and malicious, meant solely to harm or embarrass the patient.

It is also interesting to note that the hospital immediately distanced itself from the doctor, indicating that he was on his own to defend his actions and that the hospital would not defend him in any way.

Media and Hospital Marketing

Social media can be a wonderful tool to build relationships and connect with the community. Through social media, hospitals and other healthcare organizations can disseminate health information, increase credibility, and foster loyalty. However, safeguards need to be in place to ensure that patient confidentiality remains intact and that patient privacy is protected.

One of the most comprehensive guides to social media is *The Health Communicator's Social Media Toolkit,* which is published by the Centers for Disease Control and Prevention. This toolkit provides step-by-step instructions for running a positive and effective social media campaign (CDC, n.d.).

When initiating a social media campaign, nurse managers must first confirm the hospital's policies and procedures for social media. Typically, only those persons who are authorized to speak for the hospital on social media are to do so. If a nurse manager feels strongly that he or she would like to participate in social media on behalf of the organization, then the nurse manager should notify hospital administration of this desire and gain the proper clearances.

THE BOTTOM LINE

Social media is a wonderful communication tool that can allow us to reach out to people a world away; however, before posting any information on social media, always ask yourself how it would play in a courtroom. If you are in doubt … don't post!

References

Abramson, A. (2013, August 20). Chicago Doctor Accused of Posting Photos of Intoxicated Patient. *ABC News*. Retrieved from *http://abcnews.go.com/US/chicago-doctor-sued-photographing-hospitalized-intoxicated-woman/story?id = 20003303*.

Associated Press. (2015, March 10). VA Hospital Manager Caught Emailing Inappropriate Messages About Veterans. *US News & World Report*. Retrieved from *http://www.usnews.com/news/articles/2015/03/10/va-hospital-manager-caught-emailing-inappropriate-images-about-veterans*.

CDC. (n.d.). *The Health Communicator's Social Media Toolkit*. Retrieved from *www.cdc.gov/healthcommunication/ToolsTemplates/SocialMediaToolkit_BM.pdf*.

Kaplan, A.M., & Haenlein, M. Users of the world, unite! The challenges and opportunities of social media. *Business Horizons, 53*(1), 59–68. Retrieved from *http://michaelhaenlein.com/Publications/Kaplan,%20Andreas%20-%20Users%20of%20the%20world,%20unite.pdf*.

National Council of State Boards of Nursing. (2011). White Paper: A Nurse's Guide to the Use of Social Media. Retrieved from *www.ncsbn.org/11_NCSBN_Nurses_Guide_Social_Media.pdf*. Chicago.

Neporent, L. (2014, July 8). Nurse Firing Highlights Hazards of Social Media in Hospitals. *ABC News*.

Oregon Board of Nursing. (2012). *31*(1).

Wilson, K.A.C. (2012, March 7). Gresham woman banned from social networking after posting nude photo of nursing home patient on Facebook. *The Oregonian*. Retrieved from *www.oregonlive.com/gresham/index.ssf/2012/03/gresham_woman_banned_from_soci.html*.

11

Interprofessional Collaboration and Accountability

Nurse Manager Job Description

The nurse manager promotes a cooperative relationship among healthcare teams by building rapport and promoting a culture of collaboration.

Learning objectives

After reading this chapter, the participant will be able to do the following:

- Discuss the importance of teamwork in healthcare delivery
- List the four core competencies of interprofessional collaboration
- Identify the role of communication in interprofessional collaboration

Effective patient care is a team effort involving a group of people with various skills working together for the good of the patient. In the continuum of care, each healthcare professional contributes a specific and significant benefit to the patient.

When a healthcare team fails to work together, patient care suffers. For true teamwork to exist, healthcare professionals must not only understand their roles as professionals but also understand, appreciate, and respect the roles of other healthcare professionals (Bridges et al., 2011).

A new trend in healthcare education is for students to participate in interprofessional education. These students—in fields such as medicine, nursing, pharmacy, social work, physical therapy, and occupational therapy—work together to learn collaborative techniques to improve patient outcomes. As defined by the World Health Organization (WHO), interprofessional education occurs when "students from two or more professions learn about, from, and with each other to enable effective collaboration and improve health outcomes" (WHO, 2010).

There is no doubt that when these newly educated professionals enter the healthcare workplace, their interprofessional education will have a positive effect on healthcare and patient outcomes. Currently, however, much of the healthcare workforce has not yet been educated in interprofessional collaboration. These experienced staff members need to develop a greater understanding and appreciation of teamwork in healthcare. Here, the nurse manager is in a prime position to promote interprofessional collaboration and model cooperative behaviors.

WHO has defined interprofessional collaborative practice as follows:

> *When multiple health workers from different professional backgrounds work together with patients, families, carers [sic] and communities to deliver the highest quality of care.*

Promoting Interprofessional Collaboration

Nurse managers are perfectly positioned to promote cooperative relationships among healthcare professionals because they directly interact with hospital administration, the medical staff, and direct care professionals. To build cooperative relationships among these various professionals, the nurse manager must serve as a role model for teamwork, cooperation, and communication.

The core competencies of interprofessional collaboration were defined by a 2011 interdisciplinary panel in the publication *Core Competencies for Interprofessional Collaborative Practice: Report of an Expert Panel* (2011). These core competencies fall into four categories:

1. Values and ethics for interprofessional practice

2. Roles and responsibilities

3. Interprofessional communication

4. Teams and teamwork

Values and Ethics for Interprofessional Practice

In order to implement the values and ethics that are necessary for interprofessional collaboration, there must be a "mutual respect and trust" between the healthcare professionals on your unit. As stated by the core competencies expert panel noted earlier, this mutual respect must "honor the diversity that is reflected in the individual expertise each profession brings to care delivery" (2011).

The way that you as nurse manager foster mutual respect on your unit is through your own behavior: You must act with honesty and integrity toward all staff and patients on your unit. Your nursing staff looks to you for leadership and cues regarding how to interact with others, and you must take this role very seriously and always model professional behavior. There will be many times in your career when you become frustrated or angry with hospital administration or a member of the medical staff. Experiencing these feelings is perfectly normal and acceptable, but you must be very careful not to verbalize them in front of your staff. When you verbalize negative feelings about other professional groups, you devalue them in the eyes of your nursing staff.

Roles and Responsibilities

Each specific healthcare profession has its own legally defined set of practice boundaries and core competencies. "Learning to be interprofessional requires an understanding of how professional roles and responsibilities complement each other in patient-centered … care." According to the core competencies panel, legally identified boundaries between healthcare professionals contribute to safe and effective patient care and ensure that all aspects of patient care are covered (Interprofessional Education Collaborative Expert Panel, 2011).

In other chapters, we have discussed in great detail the legal roles of nurses and how those roles are defined by state and federal law. When supporting interprofessional collaborative practice, your role is to ensure that your nursing staff understands the legal roles and responsibilities of other healthcare professionals—those outside the nursing staff—and how each profession works to provide patient care within their own set of state and federal mandates.

Interprofessional Communication

In the legal arena, there are many examples in which patients were harmed due to a lack of adequate and necessary communication between professionals. When this breakdown in communication occurs, it is the patient who suffers the consequences. Often, healthcare professionals fail to speak up and share their knowledge about a patient's condition because they feel inferior or, because of hospital hierarchy, they do not believe that their opinions are valued. The core competencies panel found that overcoming these communication boundaries is essential for safe patient care (Interprofessional Education Collaborative Expert Panel, 2011).

Your role in fostering accurate communication is to continually acknowledge the contributions of each healthcare professional on your unit and to verbalize that each person, regardless of hospital hierarchy, contributes significantly to patient care. One important way to do this is by immediately addressing disrespectful behavior on your unit. When you witness a healthcare professional being disrespectful to another, you *must* address the situation. If you fail to do so, you send the message that such behavior is acceptable on your unit, and you devalue the professional who was the subject of the disrespectful behavior.

Teams and Teamwork

Teamwork requires collaboration between all professionals providing patient care. "Teamwork behaviors involve cooperating in the patient-centered delivery of care, coordinating one's care with other health professionals so that gaps, redundancies, and errors are avoided; and collaborating with others through shared problem-solving and shared decision making." The core competencies panel found that interprofessional collaboration promotes "interdependence" among professionals and encourages professionals' reliance upon one another (Interprofessional Education Collaborative Expert Panel, 2011).

This interdependence will occur only if professionals trust and value all professions in healthcare and communicate with them respectfully and consistently.

The goal is a positive patient outcome

As reported by the core competencies expert panel, there may be conflict between professionals when promoting interprofessional collaboration:

> [The potential source of conflict] is the diversity of their expertise areas and professional liabilities. Conflicts may arise over leadership, especially when status or power is confused with authority based on professional expertise. Whatever the source, staying focused on patient-centered goals and dealing with the conflict openly and constructively through effective interprofessional communication and shared problem-solving strengthen the ability to work together and create a more effective team (Interprofessional Education Collaborative Expert Panel, 2011).

The goal in promoting interprofessional communication and working through its challenges is positive patient outcomes.

The Legal Risks of Failed Interprofessional Collaboration

As mentioned earlier, more than a few lawsuits have occurred when interprofessional collaboration was not implemented or was ineffectively utilized. In discussing core competencies of interprofessional collaboration, the consistent theme is the need for professionals to *communicate* with one another. Lack of communication has resulted in numerous patient care errors and lawsuits.

The legal risks when interprofessional collaboration is not implemented and healthcare professionals do not communicate with one another have been identified in the research, with the failure to communicate as one of the leading causes of medical errors and patient harm. According to the Joint Commission, communication failures were the root factor for more than 70% of sentinel events.

Communication problems between nurses and physicians remains a safety issue for patients, and such issues must be resolved in order for interprofessional collaboration to be fully effective. Nurses continue to cite communication issues with physicians as contributing to their patient care errors. For example, nurses feel intimidated or pressured to give medications that they do not think are safe because they are unable to communicate their concerns to physicians or because they are intimidated when they do so. These nurses state that they have altered the way they handle order clarifications or medication questions because of intimidation.

Your goal as the nurse manager is to promote interprofessional collaboration through communication with and respect of all healthcare professionals. You also must ensure that your nursing staff feel secure and confident in the difficult job they are asked to perform. These two missions may often be in conflict, but you must remember that your nurses' professional expertise and experience should be respected and, when conflict arises, you must handle it in a professional and constructive manner.

References

Bridges, et al. (2011). Interprofessional collaboration: Three best practice models of interprofessional education. *Medical Education Online.* Retrieved from *www.ncbi.nlm.gov/pmc/articles/PMC3081249. 16:10.3402/meo.v16i0.6035.*

Institute for Safe Medication Practices. (2004). Intimidation: Practitioners Speak Up About this Unresolved Problem (Part 1). Retrieved from *www.ismp.org/newsletters/acutecare/ articles/20040311_2.asp.*

Interprofessional Education Collaborative Expert Panel. (2011). Core competencies for interprofessional collaborative practice: Report of an expert panel. Washington, D.C.: Interprofessional Education Collaborative, 18, 20, 22, 24. Retrieved from *www.aacn.nche.edu/education-resources/ipecreport.pdf.*

Joint Commission on Accreditation of Healthcare Organizations. (2005). The 2005 National Patient Safety Goals. Retrieved from *www.jointcommission.org/PatientSafety/National PatientSafetyGoals.*

Leonard, S., Graham, S., & Bonacum, D. (2004). The human factor: The critical importance of effective teamwork and communication in providing safe care. *Quality & Safety in Health Care.* Retrieved from *www.ncbi.nlm.nih.gov/pmc/articles/PMC1765783/pdf/v013p00i85.pdf.*

Long (2011). *Core Competencies for Interprofessional Collaborative Practice: Report of an Expert Panel.* American Association of Colleges of Nursing, American Association of Colleges of Osteopathic Medicine, American Association of Colleges of Pharmacy, American Dental Education Association, Association of American Medical Colleges, and Association of Schools of Public Health.

National Council of State Boards of Nursing. *www.ncsbn.org.*

World Health Organization. (2010). *Framework for action on interprofessional education & collaborative practice.* Geneva: World Health Organization. Retrieved from *www.who.int/hrh/resources/framework_ action/en/.*

12

Protecting Yourself and Your License

Nurse Manager Job Description

The nurse manager understands the legal implications and liabilty risk of the position and proactively prepares for potential legal challenges.

Learning objectives

After reading this chapter, the participant will be able to do the following:

- Discuss the reasons to purchase professional liability insurance
- Identify three actions a nurse must take when appearing before the disciplinary panel of a state nursing board

Even if you do everything correctly, you can still have a lawsuit filed against you. In addition to being stressful and expensive, a lawsuit can negatively affect your professional license, so it is essential that you protect that license proactively.

Sit for a minute and consider the value of your nursing license. It represents your professional identity and, most likely, provides your livelihood. Your nursing license is your property, and you must protect it in the same manner that you protect your other property interests.

State nursing boards recognize that your nursing license is a property right. According to the Kansas State Board of Nursing, "when we grant a license to practice nursing, we are granting a property right" (Kansas State Board of Nursing, n.d.). The Massachusetts Board of Registration in Nursing also identifies your nursing license as a property right, stating the following:

> *The U.S. Constitution and state administrative law provide for the due process rights of a nurse against whom a complaint is filed. The nurse is presumed innocent until proven guilty and has a constitutional right to keep his or her license (the nurse's property interest) until completion of the Board's complaint resolution proceedings (Massachusetts Board of Registration in Nursing, n.d.).*

Protecting Your Property Interest

When you appreciate the property interest you have in your nursing license, you will be more likely to take the necessary actions to protect it. In the following section, we will discuss the actions you must take to protect your nursing license in the event that a lawsuit is filed against you.

Are you protected under your employing hospital's insurance?

As nurses, we are assured that we are covered under our hospital's liability insurance and that we can depend on the hospital's policy when legal action is taken against our license. However, this belief is misleading—relying solely on the hospital's liability insurance policy can result in inadequate liability protection and, ultimately, money out of the nurse's pocket.

Your hospital has purchased liability insurance and, as a nurse, you might assume that you are fully protected under your hospital's insurance policies. However, you have no knowledge of the type of insurance your hospital carries, or whether that insurance will cover you if you are named in a lawsuit or called before your nursing board. For example, your hospital may have purchased insurance containing provisions that exclude coverage for nurses practicing outside their scope of employment. It is imperative that you buy your own professional liability insurance to protect your interests.

When a hospital defends a lawsuit, its primary interest is in protecting itself. There may be legal allegations in which the nurse's legal interests are contrary to the legal interests of the hospital. In such situations, a nurse who assumes that he or she is covered under the hospital's liability insurance will in fact be pitted *against* the hospital in legal action. In such situations, the attorney retained by the hospital's insuring agency may withdraw from representing the nurse. The nurse will then be forced to find his or her own attorney.

In addition, when the hospital defends a lawsuit based on the actions of a specific nurse, the hospital can bring an indemnity claim against the nurse to recover the damages the hospital is ordered to pay. The intention of such claims is to recoup money from those whose actions caused a lawsuit to be filed. In such a situation, without your own professional liability insurance, you would be required to indemnify the hospital from your own funds.

THE BOTTOM LINE

It cannot be stated strongly enough: Each nurse must buy an individual professional liability insurance policy.

Professional Liability Insurance

The terms of professional liability policies vary greatly, so make sure that you know what you are getting when you buy one. Generally, when a lawsuit is filed against a nurse, the insurance company will provide an attorney to represent the nurse. Most, if not all, insurance companies keep lawyers on retainer, which means that the insurance company pays the attorney a fee that guarantees that the attorney will be available to represent the insurance company's interests.

When a nurse is sued, his or her insurance company usually insists that the nurse use one of its attorneys. Doing so assures the nurse and the insurance company that the lawyer representing the claim is experienced in professional negligence litigation.

The Legal Authority of Your State Board of Nursing

Your state board of nursing has the legal authority to regulate your nursing license and practice. It is an administrative agency, bound by administrative law, statutes, and agency-made rules. Such agencies have statutory authority to carry out the specific intentions of statutes by creating rules and regulations that enforce them.

State boards of nursing are charged with protecting the citizens of their state by regulating nursing licensure, discipline, and continuing education. You must be knowledgeable of the laws under which you are expected to practice. Therefore, one of your best defenses in your daily nursing practice is knowing the rules and regulations of your state board of nursing.

The complaint process

When a complaint is made about nursing practice, the state board of nursing investigates the allegations and then, if warranted by the evidence, holds a hearing regarding the allegations. At that hearing, you will be given the opportunity to defend your practice and explain how you met the standard of care. Depending upon the procedures followed by your state board of nursing, your first face-to-face contact with the board may be an appearance before a disciplinary panel at an informal settlement conference.

Note that state nursing boards employ attorneys who work each day to enforce the nursing practice act of your state. Any action by your state board of nursing against your license is very serious, and you must treat it as such. When defending your license before the state board of nursing, you must take the following actions:

1. Contact your insurance company to notify it of the action
2. Hire an attorney (if one is not provided by your insurance company)
3. Attend the settlement conference
4. Be open, honest, and respectful with the board

If, after the hearing, the allegations against the nurse are substantiated, the state board of nursing administers disciplinary actions. These disciplinary actions vary greatly and depend upon the seriousness of the allegations.

Hire an attorney

Your state nursing board has legal representation through its staff attorneys, and these attorneys will be at the hearing to argue that you violated the nurse practice act. This means that you will need and must retain legal representation to defend your rights during the hearing. You will be anxious on the day of the hearing, and you will need a professional who is familiar with the processes of your state board to represent your best interests.

To find such an attorney, contact your state nursing association and ask them to recommend an attorney with experience representing nurses before the state board. Ideally, this attorney should have substantial administrative law experience. Contact the attorney, and ask questions to determine his or her knowledge of your state's nursing practice act, as well as the extent of his or her experience appearing before the state board of nursing. You do not want to be the attorney's first case before your state nursing board. If disciplinary actions are taken against your nursing license, the attorney will advise you regarding your appropriate recourse.

Before the hearing, meet with the attorney to practice what you will say during the hearing. Doing so is very important, because you want to know what you are going to say and how you are going to defend yourself—*before* you get in the stressful hearing situation.

Attend the hearing

Although attending the hearing is generally considered optional, it is essential that you be there. The decisions made by the disciplinary panel at the hearing influence your professional future, as well as the status of your nursing license. You *must* be involved in this process. You have a property interest in your professional license, and you don't want decisions made about that property interest without your input.

As an attorney with experience working for a state medical board, I have witnessed numerous hearings where the licensed professional chose not to attend the hearing. At these hearings, the board members questioned the professional's commitment to their profession and their desire to retain their medical license. Choosing not to attend the hearing reflects poorly on the nurse in question.

Be open, honest, and respectful with the board

Prior to holding a hearing to discuss disciplinary action against your license, the state board of nursing completes an extensive investigation into the complaint. Depending on the allegations against you, the board may have secured expert reports to establish how a reasonably prudent nurse in a similar situation would have responded.

These expert reports provide the board with additional evidence that you have violated the nursing practice act. You, too, may retain experts to testify that your nursing practice was reflective of a reasonably prudent nurse in a similar situation. If you made mistakes in your patient care, admit the mistakes and inform the board of actions taken to ensure that those mistakes do not occur a second time.

Depending on the severity of the patient outcome, boards generally give a professional a second chance when he or she accepts responsibility for mistakes. Boards expect a candid discussion about the issues. This may be difficult, especially if your actions resulted in an adverse patient outcome; however, successfully defending your license depends upon your open and honest communication.

Finally, be respectful of the board, and do not question its authority to take action against your nursing license. The board's authority over your nursing license is solidly grounded in statute, and it takes the mission of protecting citizens of its state very seriously.

THE BOTTOM LINE

Buy liability insurance!

References

Kansas State Board of Nursing. (n.d.). Position Statement on Multistate Regulation of Nurses. Retrieved from *www.ksbn.org.*

Massachusetts Board of Registration in Nursing. (n.d.). Board of Nursing Complaint Process Facts. Health and Human Services. Retrieved from *http://www.mass.gov/eohhs/gov/departments/dph/programs/ hcq/dhpl/nursing/complaint-resolution/board-of-nursing-complaint-process-facts.html.*

13

Ten Strategies
to Reduce Liability

Having read the first 12 chapters of this book, you know that, as a nurse manager, you are held to a higher level of accountability that includes responsibility not just for your own actions but also for those of your nursing staff. You know that successful nurse managers recognize the legal risks they may face and take every step available to prevent those legal issues from arising.

One frustrating aspect of the healthcare legal environment is that, even if you do everything correctly, you can *still* get sued. The bottom line is that there is no practice you can implement to *guarantee* that you will not be sued. That said, you can reduce your liability risks by keeping in mind a few practical ideas that encapsulate the best practices of the preceding chapters.

Your Top Ten Strategies

These strategies, when implemented in your daily practice as a nurse manager, will significantly reduce your liability risk:

1. Treat all your staff in the same manner

2. Follow the policies and procedures

3. Don't ignore problem employees

4. Keep your work environment safe

5. Never understaff your unit

6. Delegate within the boundaries of the law

7. Protect the patient's privacy

8. Show respect, and expect respect

9. Have each other's backs

10. Buy the insurance

❶ Treat all your staff in the same manner

In Chapter 2, "Employment Law for the Nurse Manager," we discussed state and federal laws under which you will be required to practice. These complicated and detailed laws define how you, the nurse manager, are to handle employment issues, family medical leave request, and discriminatory issues.

When you look at each of these state and federal laws, the underlying principle is that every employee should be given the opportunity to work and should be treated fairly in the work environment. To do this, you must treat all your staff in the same manner.

On first look, this may seem like a simplistic approach to the matter. However, managing your work environment with this as your guiding principle—treating all your staff in the same way—will increase your respect from the nursing staff, validate you as a nursing leader, and reduce your risk of facing a discrimination lawsuit or an employee's complaint with the EEOC.

❷ Follow policies and procedures to the letter

In your managerial role, you want to be consistent in carrying out the daily operations of your unit, and that consistency comes from always following your hospital's policies and procedures to the letter. Consistently following your facility's written policies and procedures is no less important than ensuring that your facility practices within identified professional standards and in compliance with state and federal law.

In Chapter 4, "The Legal Significance of Policies and Procedures," we discussed how the court views violations of established policies and procedures. If you find yourself in a lawsuit trying to defend actions that violated your facility's policies and procedures, you will face a difficult experience with the plaintiff's attorney. He or she will have your facility's policies and procedures in hand and will question you step by step to determine whether your nursing practice deviated from any of those written standards. If you have deviated, even minimally, it may raise doubt that you practiced within the standard of care.

It is important also to consider the benefits of consistency from the patient's viewpoint. Being admitted to the hospital is a stressful situation, and patients lose much of their autonomy in that context. One way to reduce some of the stress patients experience is to always treat them in a consistent manner—which is accomplished by following the policies and procedures outlined by your hospital.

When your nursing staff follows the policies and procedures of your hospital, they communicate to patients that "we are all on the same page here" and "we've got this covered," which, in turn, reassures the patient.

❸ Don't ignore problem employees

From the managerial perspective, you want to keep your good employees happy, and you want to encourage your problem employees to make the change to become good employees, or you need to take the legal steps necessary to terminate them from employment. When you ignore problem employees and fail to confront them on their behavior, you are reinforcing that behavior and defeating the morale of your good employees.

Consider a problem employee from the good employee's viewpoint. A good employee is the one who always shows up to work on time, has a good attitude, and "goes the extra mile" to ensure that patient care is being delivered in a safe and effective manner. When the good employee consistently observes you, the nurse manger, failing to intervene in a problem employee situation, the good employee begins to question his or her commitment to the unit and may seek employment elsewhere.

By failing to address the behavior of the problem employee, you are communicating to good employees that you do not respect them or the contributions they make to the unit. To retain your good employees, do not ignore problem employees.

From a legal perspective, ignoring the behavior of problem employees opens the door to lawsuits. Problem employees are more likely to make errors, jeopardize patient safety, and provide nursing care that is below the standard of care. If a lawsuit is filed against a problem employee, you may be questioned by the plaintiff's attorney regarding your knowledge that the problem employee had existing performance issues and how you addressed those concerns. You will have difficulty establishing that the employee in question did not have other job performance concerns, especially when those behaviors were witnessed by other members of your staff.

Clearly, your best defense is to have addressed the problem behaviors, documented your actions in the employee's personnel file, and monitored the problem employee closely.

❹ Keep your work environment safe

A commitment to workplace safety means that you must advocate for your nurses and speak to hospital administration when unsafe conditions exist. Although it may sound straightforward on the surface, advocating for safety is not always easy to manage when you consider the numerous safety issues—such as workplace violence, bloodborne pathogens, or orthopedic injuries—that confront nurses on a daily basis. Clearly, you must be diligent and continually monitor nursing safety on your unit.

Consider this issue from your own viewpoint: As a nurse and a nurse manager, you want to be safe in your workplace. When you are not safe in the workplace, your focus isn't on patient care; it is on your own safety and well-being. When your focus is taken off patient care, the patient suffers.

The same may be said about the safety of your nursing staff. If your nursing staff is constantly "looking over their shoulders" because they are concerned about their own safety, the patient care being delivered will suffer. If your nursing staff has identified a safety concern and brought it to your attention, you must consider yourself "on notice" regarding the safety concern. If a nurse is injured and files a lawsuit against the hospital, you don't want to find yourself in the position where you must testify that you knew about the safety concern but did not act to remedy it.

❺ Never understaff your unit

Nurses cannot be in two places at one time, but that is what is expected of them when a unit is understaffed. As the nurse manager, you must critically and constantly evaluate the staffing patterns on your unit and, when you identify an understaffing problem, take action right away. Immediately notify your direct supervisor of the staffing issues, and work with that person to remedy the situation as quickly as possible. As has been stated over and over in this book, make sure to document your actions to mitigate your liability.

Staffing is a delicate balance because it requires you to plan for something before it happens. This means that you must know your unit well and understand the staffing levels required to handle the patient acuity on your unit.

There will be times when your staffing decisions are challenged and times when you'll be encouraged to reduce your staffing levels due to budgetary reasons. Yes, staffing a hospital unit is a very expensive undertaking, but a lawsuit that results from understaffing will be much, much more expensive.

❻ Delegate within the boundaries of the law

Legal boundaries identify the borders and limits of nursing practice. Your charge nurses are your greatest asset when it comes to delegating within the boundaries of the law. However, for your charge nurses to serve as this asset, you must have fully communicated your position regarding staffing, and that position must be consistent with state law, nursing standards, and your facility's policies and procedures.

When it comes to delegation, make sure that your charge nurses know that you will not tolerate delegation of tasks to persons who are not legally qualified to carry out those tasks or who do not have the skills to do so. Make sure that your charge nurses know that you will not waiver on this position.

❼ Confidentiality is key

As a nurse manger, you will have access to highly confidential staff information. This confidential information will have the potential to destroy a person's reputation and ability to work on your unit if you do not handle it correctly and with the greatest of care and respect.

For example, you do not want to openly discuss or even "leak" the fact that one of your employees is HIV-positive because that information may negatively impact their working conditions and open you up to a lawsuit. That is not your information to share; that is your information to keep confidential.

When you gain confidential information about an employee, the best rule of thumb is never to share it with anyone unless, as in the case of human resources, they have a legal need to know the information. If you share it with others, you put yourself at risk of being sued for discrimination under the statutes (discussed at length in Chapter 2, "Employment Law for the Nurse Manager"). You may also face civil charges, such as slander and liable, depending on how and with whom you shared this information.

Carefully and closely guard all confidential staff information, and never make an exception to that rule.

❽ Show respect—Expect respect

We want to be respected in both our professional and personal lives. However, that does not always happen, and, in your role as nurse manager, there will be times when you are disrespected, intimidated, or spoken to in a condescending manner.

You cannot control how others treat you, but you can control how you treat others. In all that you do, do it with respect toward others. If you are disrespected by someone, do not return the behavior. Meet that disrespect with respect, and then address the offending behavior through the appropriate policies and procedures at your hospital. Do not ignore the disrespectful behavior, but handle it through the appropriate chain of command.

During your career, you also may witness disrespect that escalates to assaultive behavior. As an attorney with experience working for a state medical board, I've worked on cases where the disrespectful behavior of hospital employees crossed the line to the level of assault and battery. For example, in one case, a surgeon was brought before his state medical board for having thrown a scalpel at a surgical assistant. The physician was referred to peer review within his hospital and was disciplined by his employing hospital. The physician was also disciplined by his state medical board.

In this case, it also would have been within the surgical assistant's legal rights to file a civil suit against the physician. These types of behaviors are unacceptable in any setting, are disruptive to employee morale, and place patient safety at risk.

It bears repeating: Immediately address disrespectful behavior following the policies of your organization. Do not let it escalate.

❾ Have each other's backs

Nurses must support each other; that is all there is to it. In your hospital, seek out other nurse managers who understand your daily challenges and who will be willing to provide support when you need it.

Nursing is a difficult profession, and being a nurse manager adds to that stress. You will need support from other nurse managers you trust and with whom the information you share will be respected and your confidentiality protected. Tell them that you will offer the same, and mean it.

Protect and support each other and "have each other's backs."

❿ Buy the insurance

Last but not least … **buy the insurance**! As we have discussed in great detail, nursing managers face multiple liabilities from many fronts. When you implement risk management practices, such as those discussed in this book, your risk for a lawsuit is reduced; however, the risk never truly goes away, and you can be sued even if you do everything correctly.

You must always be prepared for a lawsuit. The primary way to do so is to buy the insurance. Most likely, you will never need it, but on the off chance that you do, it will be the greatest security you have when facing legal allegations against your nursing license.

Legal Glossary

Legal Terms and Definitions	
Term	**Definition**
Breach	A violation of a law, standards of care, or policies and procedures
Causal connection	In nursing, the direct relationship of a nurse's action or inaction on a patient outcome
Code of ethics	A set of established standards that guides the moral code of an organization or an individual
Conscientious objection	When a nurse objects to a treatment or intervention based on the individual nurse's moral or ethical belief system
Cue recognition	The ability to identify verbal or physical signs that a person may become violent
Damage	Loss or injury to a person or property

Duty of care	A legal obligation the nurse has to his or her patients. Generally, this duty arises when the nurse accepts care of the patient.
Duty to report (ethical)	The nurse's requirement to report practices or situations that challenge his or her moral compass—when something doesn't "feel right"
Duty to report (legal)	The requirement to report illegal practices or situations as defined by state nursing boards/state law
Foreseeable result	An outcome that a reasonably prudent nurse could predict based on experience or education
Lateral violence	Peer-on-peer hostile, aggressive, or violent behavior
Lawsuit	Any proceeding by a party or parties against another in a court of law
Negligence	Conduct that falls below the standard established by law for the protection of others against unreasonable risk or harm
No-tolerance policy	An infraction, no matter how minimal, of an established standard will be deemed a violation of that standard and will be punishable
Patient abandonment	After accepting the care of a patient, terminating the nurse-patient relationship without reasonable notice, without transferring care to a qualified nursing professional, and/or without being relieved of that responsibility by the nursing supervisor
Policies and procedures	Formalized written principles under which a hospital manages its organization. Answers the question, "How do we do things in this hospital?"
Policies and procedures (other media)	Videos or training materials that may establish practices in a hospital and may be held in court to be principles under which a hospital is managed
Policies and procedures (unwritten)	Verbal understandings, such as verbal physician orders, that may establish practices in a hospital and be held in court to be principles under which a hospital is managed

Prima facie	A clear-cut, unambiguous cause, recognized "at first glance" with no need to look further for additional causes
Professional malpractice	Negligence committed by a person when acting within his or her professional capacity
Proximate cause	The potential for harm is foreseeable
Reasonably prudent nurse benchmark for standard of care	What a nurse with similar experiences and education would do in similar circumstances
Retaliation	Negative and illegal actions against a person for having become a whistleblower. Such actions may include work assignment changes, threats from management, or termination of employment.
Standard of care in nursing practice	What a nurse with similar experiences and education would do in similar circumstances
Whistleblower	A nurse shares information that his or her employer is violating federal and/or state laws, or the nurse knows that the employer is engaging in practices that place the public or patients at risk. The nurse reports that information to the appropriate authority, thus "blowing the whistle" on his or her employer.
Whistleblower protection program	State and federal laws that protect the whistleblower from negative and illegal retaliation
Workplace bullying	Nurse-on-nurse hostility and aggression that occurs between healthcare professionals
Workplace violence	Aggression, harassment, physical threats, or assault against nurses perpetrated by patients, hospital visitors, or other hospital staff